POP UP ON TI

A GENERAL PRACTICE MEMOIR

EUGENE HUGHES

ABOUT THE AUTHOR

Eugene Hughes was born at the Lourdes hospital in Drogheda, Eire, in 1956. Pierce Brosnan was also born in this hospital, but that is where the similarity ends. Eugene grew up in the north of England, before going to Guy's Hospital medical school in 1974. He qualified in 1979, and began a series of hospital posts before ending up in general practice on the south coast. His interest in diabetes led to him being a founder member of the Primary Care Diabetes Society UK, and he was chairman of Primary Care Diabetes Europe for four years. He has published books on diabetes, articles, editorials, and learned papers.

After thirty years in general practice, he retired in 2015, and lives quietly with his wife and dog (Hugo). They have two sons and three grandchildren. He does not have homes in New York, or the south of France.

To my parents, my wife, and my children, who believed in me.

'The art of medicine consists of amusing the patient while nature cures the disease.'

Voltaire

Contents

Introduction

The title of this book was inspired by a comment made by my elderly mother.

'Have you ever noticed how often doctors use the word 'pop'?' she asked.

It is true.

'I'm just going to pop this needle in your arm.'

'I'll pop in and see you next week.'

'We'll soon pop this one out.' (sebaceous cyst of scalp).

'We'll soon pop this one out.' (recalcitrant baby).

'I'll just pop this in.' (finger).

'I'll just pop this in.' (fiendish metal instrument).

'Why don't you pop behind this curtain...

...pop your things off...

..and pop up on the couch.'

Whilst you will have no possible occasion to doubt the veracity of my account, there are some individuals who might take offence with regard to their inclusion. Therefore, in order to preserve anonymity, I have replaced some of the surnames with the names of towns and villages picked randomly from The New Shell Guide to England (1981). Well, almost randomly. Not even the most troublesome patient, nor the most abhorrent consultant deserves to be saddled with the name of Slough or Staines.

I did once know a Dr Hull once. And a Dr Leeds, for that matter.

Just saying.

Oh, and I hope you don't mind, but I will refer to patients as *patients*, not as *clients* or *customers*, or, God help us, *service users*. One of the problems with our ailing NHS is the profusion of managers, and their inevitable abuse of the English language - manager-speak. Each reorganisation brings a new wave of targets and terminology, which I detest. For the same reason, you will not find me *pushing the bloody envelope, thinking out of the box, or being in symbiosis.*

In the beginning

In the early years after qualifying, I might find myself at a dinner party, or a drinks evening, where the subject of conversation would inevitably turn to 'What made you want to become a doctor in the first place?'

At such a point in time, I would be tempted to strike a pose, heavy with gravitas, and reply, 'I have always been fascinated by the human condition' or 'It came from a deep seated need to be a healer' or, even worse 'I suppose you could call it my vocation in life.'

The true answer is somewhat more prosaic.

I went to a fairly crummy Roman Catholic comprehensive school in the north of England. One day we were warned to expect 'something special'. This came in the form of a stout balding priest from Belfast who expounded at great length on the virtues of priesthood. He concluded his talk with a dire warning about the impending world shortage of priests, and exhorted us all to look deep within our souls and listen to God's call. I looked deep into my soul. I heard His call.

That evening, as we sat around the kitchen table, I announced to my parents that I was going to be a priest. I could sense a slight quivering of my mother's upper lip, as her Irish heritage tugged at her heartstrings. Oh, the joy, the pride.., the heavenly reward....

My father hardly looked up from his shepherd's pie and peas.

'Don't be so bloody daft.'

After due deliberation, (about ten minutes), I concluded that he was probably right and that I should instead become a doctor.

When this desire was communicated to the careers teacher at the fairly crummy school, a chain of events was set in motion which effectively sealed my fate.

This school (now thankfully demolished) had, in its brief history, only sent one previous gifted individual to medical school. I was to be the second, and they would move Heaven and Earth to ensure that it came to pass.

Thus, my 'O' level and 'A' level choices were predetermined. I had been fairly good at French and wanted to take it at 'A' level as well as the standard physics, chemistry and biology. No – it would be a distraction. *Tant pis.*

I was even warned that my social life was another distraction, and that I was seeing my girlfriend too often (once a week!).

And obviously, being Head Boy would look good on the application form. There were much better candidates, but a 'democratic' vote was taken – the same sort of democracy you will encounter in central African countries – and I was duly elected. So, sorry Paul S. and Nick R.

I was told to put a London medical school at the top of my preferred choices, and inferior provincial medical schools in the other slots. They'd like that.

It all worked. I received an invitation for an interview.

The interview.

I walked past sombre, marble busts of the great and the good, and took my seat in a suitably sombre, wood panelled office across the table from three suitably sombre interviewers.

I had had the benefit of multiple rehearsals at the crummy school, but I had an alternative strategy.

I was going to lie through my teeth.

'It says here that you write poetry. Have you had any published?'

'Yes, I had a couple of northern dialect poems published in *Lancashire Life.*' Lie.

'What interests you about a medical career?'

'I have spent some time volunteering in my local hospital, and have been able to see the workings of the NHS first-hand.' Big lie.

'I also asked my own GP if I could spend some time in the practice to gain a greater understanding of patients' needs.' Bigger lie.

'And, finally, why have you chosen this particular medical school?'

'Because it is the finest in the world, and I see no point in settling for second best.' Possibly true, but delivered with such conviction, I even believed it myself.

Two weeks later, I received an offer of a place, with the proviso that I achieved 3 'C' grades in my 'A' levels. These days, 4 'A' grades or higher would be the starting point. The grades I achieved then would nowadays possibly guarantee me a future as a laboratory technician.

Medical school

Day 1

One hundred and twenty fresh-faced, eager, brand new medical students sit in rapt attention in the historic anatomy lecture theatre in late September. The dean sweeps in majestically and takes his place behind the lectern.

'Good morning students.' Dramatic pause. 'You have been given the privilege of studying medicine at the greatest institute in the world. You will have access to the finest teachers, the best facilities and two hundred years of history. Like your predecessors, you will go on to be eminent professors, to undertake ground-breaking research, and above all, to carry our good name forward into the next generation. And if you fail, there's always general practice.'

OK, so that might not have been verbatim, but it was certainly implied, and continued to be implied until the last day of the final year. This was reflected in the paucity of lectures and training in any aspect of general practice, and the measly eight weeks of attachments in the clinical years.

We knew our place. If family medicine was to be the chosen direction, it was clearly for the less able, the less ambitious, the second rate. Interestingly, about 75% of that particular intake ended up in general practice. Must have been a bad year for the finest institution in the world.

Day 2

Don't worry, I am not going to go through the next five years one day at a time. Quite the opposite, in fact. I do not intend to spend too much time recounting the details of this hilarious / heart-breaking / stressful / enchanting period of my life. Partly because I would doubt the accuracy of such an account, blurred as the edges would be by beer, tiredness, the passage of time and a sprinkling of urban myth.

But, on the second day...

I was sitting in a physiology lecture, and finding it hard to concentrate, or indeed understand what was being imparted to me by the enthusiastic figure at the front. To be honest, I felt a bit bewildered, a bit lonely, a bit homesick. If this was day 2, then there were another ten weeks till the end of term, then another two terms, then another 4 years. The future stretched away from me, an infinite, terrifying void.

'You getting any of this?' The student to my left looked bored and was doodling on his notepad.

I shook my head.

'Fancy a pint, then?'

The very thought of drinking beer at lunchtime was thrilling enough, so I agreed. He introduced himself as Al, and there began a friendship that would last for decades. We even ended up in practice in adjacent towns. Al was different.

He had had sex 88 times. Yes, he counted.

He drank pints of beer at lunchtime.

He had a handlebar moustache.

He was cool.

On the other hand;

I was a virgin.

I drank a half of bitter shandy occasionally.

I wore sports jackets.

He took me under his wing, and tried to cure me of all the above afflictions.

After the first term, he convinced me to move out of my grotty bedsit, and share a flat with him. This worked well because I was good at anatomy and he was good at biochemistry, so we were able to prop each other up in our weakest subjects. It also led to a good deal of beer drinking. The other residents in the converted Victorian terraced house we called home were two Australian sports teachers, a lesbian couple who looked like Little and Large, and a miserable cow called Germaine who couldn't stand the sight of us. The feeling was mutual. Germaine had a fat greasy boyfriend who parked his Ford Capri outside the flats. On Thursday evenings, the two Aussies and the two aspiring doctors would go out for the evening. Four pints of Guinness later, we would call in at the chippy. Our meandering route home was timed to perfection so the last chip was eaten at the exact moment we arrived at the Ford Capri, allowing us to spear the chip papers on the car aerial, before disappearing into the flat in a fit of very childish giggles.

And I still regret giving him the 'kitty' to go and get the week's shopping after he had had a couple of beers. He came back with two bottles of Southern Comfort and two packets of Garibaldi biscuits.

What else can I say about the next few years?

I worked hard, but excelled at nothing.

I met my wife to be.

We went to several of the legendary Pepys Road parties.

Finals came rushing towards us at a terrifying pace.

A part of the final examination in medicine involves a case study with a real patient. You have a set time to take a history, examine the patient, formulate a diagnosis, then face a grilling from a consultant about your findings. My progress towards becoming a qualified doctor was given a huge boost when the patient said 'I'm not supposed to tell you anything, but you look like a nice young man, so I've got Cushing's disease.'

I passed.

And so it was that a short time later I found myself in the corridor of the medical school where a neatly typed list has been affixed to the wall, anxiously scrolling down to find my name. After qualification, new doctors have to do a 'pre-registration year', usually consisting of six months in general medicine and six months in general surgery, before you are a 'proper' doctor i.e. registered with the General Medical Council. The prestige jobs, the ones in the medical school and its attached hospitals, go to the best candidates, or those whose parents are consultants, or those who have been painfully obsequious. I wasn't truly expecting one of those, obviously. I found my name and followed the line along to find out where I had been allocated. I sort of recognised the name of the town, but had to ask someone exactly where it was. I was going to spend the next year of my life, and the first year of married life, in a small seaside town on the south coast.

House jobs

My first 'house' job was in geriatrics. These days, it is referred to as 'elderly medicine' or some such term. In those days, it was the pits. Not so, however, in my hospital. Two excellent consultants, clearly ahead of their time, had created a philosophy of care that treated all the patients as though they were 50 year olds in an acute medical setting. Negativity was outlawed. All necessary tests and investigations were to be done, and the best treatment offered. I learned more in that job than in the rest of my training.

One of the consultants had the unfortunate habit of dictating his notes at the foot of the patients bed, during the ward round. He said that it aided clarity. It certainly did, for the patient as well as the junior hospital staff, as he boomed into the Dictaphone.

'Mabel Johnson, age 88. Problem number 1 – heart failure. Problem number 2 – renal failure. Problem number 3 – brain failure. Problem number 4 – carcinoma of the bladder.' I'm all for freedom of information, but there are limits.

The other consultant was an exceptionally well dressed Greek Cypriot, focussed, punctual, precise. On one ward round, he asked the ward sister 'And is Mrs. Jones having a proper diet?' 'Yes doctor', she replied 'this morning she was incontinent of faeces in her bed, then she took a spoon and ate it all up.' His Mediterranean complexion took on a greenish tinge.

Another patient told me how she had been run over by a bus when she was a small girl. 'That must have been dreadful' I remarked. 'Yes it was, as all four horses went over me.'

My surgical job involved working for three consultant surgeons. One was an aged, curmudgeonly sort who looked like a farmer, and who used sterilised lengths of fishing line to sew up surgical wounds to save the NHS money. Another was a thin, wheedling guy who found fault with everything. The scalpels weren't sharp enough, someone had given him the wrong needle or the wrong swab. It was rumoured that he had thrown one of my predecessors out of the theatre for asking 'How would you like your stitches cut today, sir, too short or too long.?' It could have been worse. One of my colleagues in a nearby town worked for a rather large surgeon, a bon viveur who had earned the title of 'the butcher'. With good reason. At the end of a seemingly routine operation he would casually announce 'we seem to have nicked the spleen, sister, could you get me a spleen kit?', or 'we seemed to have nicked the small bowel, sister, could you open another surgical pack?' Thus the simple operation became more complicated, and some patients left the theatre with much less of their anatomy than they bargained for.

The hospital training posts

The posts in my particular package were – paediatrics, obstetrics, general medicine and psychiatry.

Obstetrics

I delivered the requisite number of babies, about 30 in total.

I became an expert in episiotomy repair. An episiotomy is a cut made in the vaginal opening to facilitate the delivery of the baby's head if things are progressing too slowly for the baby's good. It sounds barbaric, but often it is done to prevent a nasty tear in the vaginal walls and opening – this is uncontrolled, and can lead to difficulties with urinary and bowel continence in years to come, so the surgical option is preferred (although there is a vigorous ongoing debate about medical intervention versus 'natural' childbirth). If the decision is made to perform the episiotomy, local anaesthetic is injected into the lower part of the vaginal opening, and a cut is made with scissors to enlarge the opening. Hopefully, everything then proceeds smoothly, the baby arrives, followed by the placenta, followed by the tears and general hullabaloo. When everyone has had a chance to hold the baby, and all the bowls, towels, and paraphernalia have been cleared away, it is time to repair the damage that the scissors, or mother nature has wreaked on the nether regions of the new mother.

This involves placing the mother's legs in an undignified position on stirrups (many women will laugh at the very idea that any dignity remains after what they have just been through). The doctor then sits on a stool between these legs, facing the task in hand, and attempts to recreate the beautiful vagina that God had bestowed in the first place. This is not always easy, as the anatomy has been distorted by swelling, the presence of the local anaesthetic, bleeding and so on. Often it requires several layers of stitches to create the perfect, aesthetic, anatomically correct, and secure result. Most junior doctors rapidly acquire this proficiency.

On one occasion, it was the wife of one of my colleagues on the same GP rotation who was in the stirrups. Delicacy dictates that a senior doctor would be called to do the necessary. Unfortunately, he was detained in theatre on a complicated and lengthy case. The options were limited – wait for several hours, or allow yours truly to step into the (literal) breach.

'Oh, for God's sake, just get on with it.' I duly obliged. So it was that someone whose face I was used to seeing across a dinner party table was now presenting a rather different part of her body to me. I prayed that this would be one of my finest surgical works of art.

It being a small hospital, however, word soon got out, and for several weeks, smutty comments circulated in the doctor's mess, mostly centring on whether the husband of the poor woman had slipped me a tenner to put an extra stitch in.

I was on the ward one day when a new patient was being admitted by my registrar, a cheerful but forgetful Sri Lankan. He had finished taking the history and examining the patient, had swept back the curtains, and was making his way down the ward, when it struck him that he had missed a vital question in the history-taking. He turned and shouted down the ward, 'Oh, I forgot to ask - when was the last time you had sexual intercourse?'

On the last day of my attachment, the registrar was performing a forceps delivery, when the consultant made an uncharacteristic appearance. 'What's going on here?' he said, nodding in my direction 'why isn't he doing this?'

'Because I haven't done one before.'

'You mean to tell me that you have worked for me for six months, and haven't done a single forceps delivery?' He was less than pleased.

'Today is my last day. I will never have to undertake this procedure in my life. I don't think it is fair to attempt to place two large metal blades round a baby's little head in order to prove a point.'

He stormed out of the room. However, he did 'sign me off' for the attachment.

And, just as importantly, I took and passed the DRCOG exam. Tick. One down.

Paediatrics.

Of all the doctors, surgeons, professors, and allied professionals who have made a significant impact on my medical career, few stand out in my mind as much as my paediatrics consultant, the wonderful, kindly Dr. Jones. A softly spoken, mild-mannered gentleman, he was compassionate, knowledgeable, experienced, and loved. Paediatrics might have been my chosen direction in medicine were it not for the extreme difficulty in making it up the ladder, consultant posts effectively being 'dead men's shoes.' I resolved to take the DCH, not only to tick another box, but because I loved the speciality, and felt I could bring the extra learning and experience into my future general practice. When he learned of my intentions, Dr Jones presented me with *Nelson's textbook of paediatrics*, a tome the size of six Argos catalogues stuck together. Most of my contemporaries were using *The Ladybird Guide to Paediatrics*, or something similar. I devoured the book, learning all the obscure syndromes and conditions. I passed. Another tick.

One of the conditions well known to *Nelson*, and indeed, any medical practitioner, is *pyloric stenosis*. This typically affects babies of around six weeks of age, and is caused by a thickening of the muscle at the bottom of the stomach. The baby presents with intractable vomiting, sometimes so forceful it is referred to as 'projectile', the stomach contents being hurled spectacularly across a room, or an unsuspecting individual.

These days, the diagnosis would be confirmed by a scan. In those days, we were trained to gently probe the stomach area of the scrawny, wailing child to feel the thickened muscle. A tricky procedure, difficult to learn. When presented with such a case, I would summon Dr Jones. He would patiently sit the baby on his lap, and his experienced fingers would go to work.

'I think you had better notify the surgeons', he would say. The surgeons would never question his call, theatres would be organised. He was never wrong. Clinical skills that are perhaps confined to the history books in this age of defensive, technology-based medicine.

I was also introduced to the acronym FLK, standing for 'funny looking kid'. This was in no way derogatory, it simply called upon your clinical skills and aptitude. If you were confronted with a rather strange story, and the child in front of you looked 'funny' – maybe the ears were a bit low-set, maybe the hairline looked different – you should start to think of rare congenital syndromes or metabolic conditions. It served me well for the rest of my junior hospital days, and into general practice, where rare things do occur, albeit rarely.

Psychiatry

My psychiatry post was a doddle.

From 9.00 a.m. to 5 p.m. I was in charge of the day hospital. Most of the patients were regular attenders, some came most days, others one or two days a week. Occasionally there would be a new recruit, or a discharge.

The patients included;

Frank, a married, retired railway worker in his 60s who suffered from the most profound, immobilising depressive state that I have ever witnessed. His life consisted of wading through black treacle day after day without any relief. He arrived promptly at nine, sat in abject misery, the black clouds almost visible above his head, and left at five when his wife came to collect him. Everything had been tried – talking therapies, medication, even ECT – all to no avail.

Wendy, a nervous woman in her 40s who was scared of everything. She had disabling anxiety, no self-confidence, no life to speak of.

Laura, a pretty girl in her twenties, who had a family history of a progressive neurological disease with a distressing prognosis. As there was, at the time, no test to determine carriers of the condition, she was forced to live with the uncertainty. She could not plan a marriage, children, a career, for fear that she would start to develop symptoms in her thirties. My consultations with her centred around trying to find reasons why she should not end her life now rather than put up with years of fear and dread.

Malcolm, a 'burned-out' schizophrenic who entertained the group with his outbursts.

Shirley, a manic-depressive lady in her 50s. During her manic phases, she would buy jumpers. During her depressive swings, she would ruminate about what to do with the hundreds of jumpers of all shades which filled every room in the house.

 My job was to monitor their progress, occasionally adjust the medication, and to write copious notes for the weekly meeting with the consultant, Dr Dunsmore. He was a short, fidgety man who always wore a grey three-piece suit. He also suffered from a mild degree of OCD, so it became the weekly entertainment to wind him up. During our meetings, he would occasionally leave the room, affording me the opportunity to make slight adjustments to the layout of the desktop. Move his coffee an inch to the right, rotate his pen through 45 degrees, slide the top sheet of his notes up a bit. On his return, there would be a rapid appraisal, an accusatory glare, then a few moments of furtive rearranging before we could proceed.

The other element of this post was the occasional commitment to the on-call rota for the large regional hospital 8 miles away. I would drive there, pick up a pager, and retire to the bar where I could enjoy a couple of pints and watch TV. Every now and then, I would be paged to authorize a sedative, or a change of dose, but this did not even require me to leave the bar. Rarely, I would have to assess and admit a patient who had been referred by a GP, social services, or the police. One such patient arrived late at night, and I arranged to see him in the deserted outpatients department. We sat in a small consulting room, and I opened with 'Why have you been brought here to see me?'

'I keep hearing voices telling me to kill people' was his stark reply. I realised at that point that I was quite alone in a remote part of the hospital, sitting behind a desk, and my only route of escape was the door, in front of which was sitting my homicidal maniac. Employing all the negotiating skills at my disposal, I managed to persuade him to accompany me to the ward, hoping all the while that he had failed to notice the thin sheen of perspiration that adorned my forehead, and hoping even more that a carefully concealed knife was not about to ruin my evening.

Two weeks before the end of this attachment, Frank waltzed into the day hospital and announced that he was cured of his depression. He had suddenly felt the clouds lift, the sun had come out, and he was back to his old self after five long years of suffering. No reason or explanation could be found, but we all went home feeling a little bit lighter that evening.

General Medicine

I was now a *Senior* house officer. That meant I had more responsibility and a bit more kudos. It also meant that I had a junior house officer to do all the mundane tasks, and was eligible to undertake more complicated procedures. These days, any serious investigation is governed by algorithms, health and safety, clinical governance. This is supposed to ensure that the same procedure, whether carried out in Penzance or Perth, will be performed to the same exacting standards. A good idea in principle, but we know from recent newspaper headlines that this is not the case. In my day, we still adhered to the 'see one, do one, teach one' philosophy. So it was that I routinely undertook procedures which would now be the premise of registrars and consultants. For example, in increasing order of scariness;

Lumbar puncture

Purpose – to determine whether an individual has meningitis

Procedure – the patient lies on their side. A long needle is inserted into the middle of the lower back and advanced between the vertebrae until the membrane surrounding the spinal cord is reached .It is then further advanced, a millimetre at a time until this membrane is punctured. The cerebrospinal fluid (the fluid around the spinal cord) is measured for pressure, and a sample taken for analysis.

Potential problems – there is a 5 millimetre leeway between puncturing the membrane and sticking a large needle into the spinal cord itself. Whilst you may get away without any serious damage, the patient will not thank you for the excruciating pain they will experience at that point.

Oh, and you could introduce bacteria, catastrophically causing the infection you were trying to detect.

Liver biopsy

Purpose – to obtain a sample of liver tissue for analysis, to make an exact diagnosis of the pathological process involved.

Procedure – the patient is given a small injection of local anaesthetic to numb the skin. They are then asked to breathe out and hold their breath. This is designed to reduce the size of the lung to enable you to get at the liver. Then, before they dare to breathe in again, you thrust a covered needle into their side, take a biopsy, then take it out again. How long can **you** hold your breath when breathing out? Precisely.

Potential problems – the patient might breathe in, presenting your biopsy apparatus with a nicely inflated lung. You might also biopsy anything else that gets in the way, including large blood vessels. These risks are lampooned in the old medical joke about the pathology report announcing 'this sample shows skin, pleura, lung, diaphragm, gall bladder, liver and pancreas. Is it a biopsy or a shish kebab?' Laugh, you might. Just don't get liver disease.

The insertion of a 'central line'

Purpose - To enable an intravenous infusion (think of a 'drip') to be established in seriously ill individuals who need large volumes of fluid rapidly because they are in a state of profound collapse. Sometimes used for giving chemotherapy or other drugs.

Procedure – the patient is placed head down, with face turned away from you (they really would not want to watch). The doctor stands at the head of the patient, feels around for landmarks like the clavicle (collar bone), then inserts a long wide-bore needle into the neck aiming downwards and towards the nipple. (I'm guessing this is why Scaramanga never had it done, but that's one for the James Bond aficionados to ponder). You are aiming for the internal jugular vein, which thankfully is a large vein, but it unhelpfully sits beside the carotid artery. If you hit the wrong one, you will know about it.

Potential problems – these days, this procedure is carried out under ultrasound guidance. Back in the day, it was more 'hit and hope' (not exactly, I never witnessed any catastrophies). But that area of the neck is populated with a bunch of interesting structures.

Chest drain

Purpose - To drain fluid from around the lung, or sometimes to allow air to escape from a punctured lung.

Procedure – you find a space between the ribs at the side of the chest, put a little local anaesthetic into the skin, then shove a large metal spike, sheathed in a plastic tube, about the diameter of a small leek (no pun intended) into the chest cavity. Once in the right place, the metal spike is removed, leaving the plastic tube to do the draining.

Potential problems – you are probably OK if you are going into the right lung. Coming from the left side, you might encounter an annoying large obstacle called the heart. It is possible to stick your large spike straight into one of the ventricles. I have known one instance when this occurred. The doctor, a consultant anaesthetist no less, had the presence of mind to leave the spike where it was, call for a heart surgeon, and hand the patient over, for the hole to be repaired.

My registrar at the time was not given to levity, jokes or japes. Which was fine, because he was very supportive, and did his fair share of the work. One day, he emerged from behind a curtained-off patient on the ward, and said 'I think it would be helpful if you assessed this patient.' I detected the merest upturning of his mouth as he left the ward.

'Good morning, I'm Dr Hughes, just here to go through the details. And your name?'

'Bill Johnson.'

'OK, Mr Johnson, so you've been admitted today, is that right?'

'Yes, doctor.'

'So, what seems to be the trouble?'

'I can't ginny ganny.'

'You can't what?'

'Well, when I ginny the ganny, I just could not ginny ganny.'

'Tell me your date of birth.'

'Twelfth of April, doctor.'

'And your address?'

'Number 27 ginny ganny, that's ginny ganny, ginny ganny, Birmingham.'

The poor man had suffered a stroke affecting his speech centre. I have no idea whether he thought he was making sense, or whether he was distressed at his ability to express himself.

He made a full recovery and went back to his home in ginny ganny, though he later moved to Wales, a sort of prophylactic measure, I suppose, in the event of a relapse.

Junior doctors, long hours, workload, and bullying

Anyone who has read the excellent *'This is going to hurt'* by Adam Kay will be completely familiar with the working conditions for junior doctors in the 1980s and 1990s. I am pleased to say that things have now changed dramatically, partially in response to the European Working Time Directive, which limits the number of hours that doctors can work in a given time. I understand that it is now 48 hours per week, and there are additional rules about the length of a shift. This is a welcome change, and there are penalties for Health Trusts which break the rules. This can lead to paradoxically ridiculous situations. One of my friends, a senior registrar in Paediatrics, was working on the ward one evening, putting up a drip on a new-born baby. The consultant appeared, and bellowed,

'What do you think you are doing?'

'Just putting up this drip, then I'm off for the evening.'

The consultant pointed to his watch and pointed to the door.

'Out. Out NOW. I'll finish this. Can't risk anyone seeing you here after hours.'

Ludicrous, but of course we now live in a world where medical knowledge and common sense are subjugated to the whims of managers. No wonder doctors are stampeding out of the NHS and heading to Canada and New Zealand.

But let us return to the 1980s for an instant. Junior doctors worked a nominal 40 hour week, plus overtime. The overtime was calculated in UMTs – units of medical time. Each UMT was 4 hours, so if the job description mentioned 16 UMTs, it meant that, in addition to your original 40 hours, you worked 4 x 16 = 64 hours on call. Now, of course, some of that time was sitting around, even sleeping, but always prepared to be up and functioning as soon as the dreaded bleep went off. For some jobs, you were unlucky to be disturbed much in the night, others, like obstetrics, it was a certainty. Babies don't elect to be born between the hours of 9.00 to 5.00. So an on-call weekend would start with a ward round at 8.00 on Friday morning, and finish at 5.00 on Monday evening. Doctors were unsurprisingly exhausted, and prone to making mistakes. Almost invariably, vigilant nursing staff would spot errors, and come to the rescue of a drooping house officer who needed practical or psychological support.

And to add insult to injury, UMTs were paid at a fraction of the normal hourly rate.

When I was a junior surgical house officer, one of my duties was to admit patients under the oral surgeons, people who required an anaesthetic for a difficult dental procedure, such as complicated wisdom tooth removal. One day, I became one of those patients. My wisdom teeth were pointing at an awkward angle, and crowding out the rest of my teeth, so they had to come out. Unfortunately, there was no-one to cover me on that day, as no locum had been found by the powers that be. I therefore checked myself into the ward, examined my heart and lungs, and prescribed my own pre-med (the lovely jab you get to make you drowsy before the actual anaesthetic.) All this is absolutely forbidden under modern medical practice, as indeed it probably was in those days. To make matters worse, as I lay there in a hazy bliss, the nurses were coming up to my bed, and asking me to sign drug charts for the other patients.

I did not encounter much in the way of bullying, though some consultants could be unpleasant just for the sake of it. Pomposity was the rule, being humiliated on the ward was commonplace. One of my peers had a different experience. She was asked by her consultant to 'clerk in' his private patients in a different part of the hospital. When she replied that it wasn't part of her job description, with the implication that the fat lazy slob should be earning the huge fee he was charging, she was simply and pointedly told that it was the responsibility of the consultant to 'sign off' her attachment, and she could choose to repeat the whole six months if she preferred.

Anaesthetics

The year passed quickly. After your twelve month stint, you are supposed to feel confident to do most things on the ward. I didn't feel particularly ready to inflict myself on the general public at that time, so I took up the offer of doing anaesthetics for a year at the same hospital. Anaesthetics has been described as '95% boredom, 5% sheer bloody panic'. It is an appropriate description. Under the watchful eye of the ever-patient, funny, compassionate Dr. Thompson, I quickly learned the basics. After the first few weeks, I was doing my own cases. After a few months, I would take solo charge of a whole operating list, and do on-call duties unassisted. There were moments of sheer bloody panic, but senior colleagues were always quickly on the scene, and I was aided considerably by the marvellous ODAs – Operating Department Assistants – who knew everything and could get you out of any deep hole.

One of my duties was to make regular visits to the Intensive Care Unit. A four-bedded unit, it was often empty, or transiently occupied by a patient who needed stabilising after major surgery. I was therefore shocked to arrive for my early morning round to see all four beds occupied – it had been empty the previous evening. The dark demeanour of the nursing staff alerted me that something was seriously wrong. My shock deepened when I recognised one of the patients as a colleague from the orthopaedic department. Then it dawned on me that all four occupants of Intensive Care were my colleagues. It transpired that they had been for an evening out, and had been involved in an horrific car accident. One of them was paralysed from the neck down, the others all had multiple injuries. Dark days followed, necessary surgery performed, slow recoveries made. Incredibly, they all returned to medical careers. The paraplegic doctor was forced to forsake his career in orthopaedics, but retrained as a psychiatrist.

Another sobering aspect of Intensive Care was the eventual realisation that recovery was never going to happen. Patients who were brain dead, and being kept alive by ventilators, drips, artificial feeds. The time would come when a decision would have to be made. In consultation with the families, senior consultants would decide that the time had come to withdraw supportive measures – 'switch the patient off'. The law required that the patient was examined by two different specialists, who had to independently agree to the process. They would sign the necessary paperwork, but it was left to the junior staff to see to the technical details - including switching off the ventilator. You cannot possibly conceive what this feels like. The nursing staff, who have shown professionalism and dedication, are now forced to watch as you disconnect wires, unplug monitors, take down drips, and turn the ventilator off. It is hard to walk the length of the treatment room with half a dozen pairs of eyes boring into your soul. They know it's not your fault, but no words are exchanged.

The consultant staff thought that I would continue my career in anaesthetics, so they encouraged me to take the Diploma of Anaesthetics, (DA) – the first stage in my journey up the ladder. I agreed to do so, even though, by now, I was feeling that my future lay in general practice. Teaching sessions were arranged, study leave granted. A few weeks before I was due to take the exam, my father collapsed and died at the young age of 51. I was devastated. I returned to my job after compassionate leave, but I was a changed man. I couldn't be bothered to take the diploma examination, I was withdrawn, irritable. One day, I overheard Dr. Thompson consoling some young junior house officer whom I had just ripped into for some trivial oversight. 'He's not himself', he told him, 'his father died recently'. I realised I needed to move on, sort myself out. I apologised to any colleagues who had had to endure my misplaced outbursts, I took, and passed, the DA. However, I was also ready to move on in my career.

But, over those eighteen months, I had been transformed. By the end of my tenure, I was ready for anything. I could take control of any medical emergency, from heart attacks to catastrophic haemorrhage, I could put a drip up anywhere, in any patient, at any time. I could anaesthetise kids, grownups, the elderly, the nearly dead. I was superman. Now I just needed a GP training post.

In the early 1980s, competition for these three year training schemes was at its most intense. I therefore spent about six months travelling round the country, attending interview after interview, suffering huge disappointments, until finally, one wonderful afternoon, in a town in the west Midlands, someone said the magic words 'You are the successful candidate.'

GP training

GP training involves a three year scheme, usually comprising a year in a training practice, divided into two six month stints, plus four other attachments of six months each, typically including obstetrics, paediatrics, and others such as dermatology, rheumatology and so on. At the end of three years, providing you have kept your nose clean, you are awarded the Joint Certificate, and can look for a post in general practice. It is possible to create your own scheme, but most people opted for the 'ready-made' package. As I have mentioned, competition for the schemes was intense, but this was as nothing compared to the nightmare of finding your dream job at the end of it. Let us not forget, that you were likely to be spending the rest of your working life in your chosen practice, probably about 40 years. Moving practices, though now commonplace, was frowned upon, and reflected badly on your commitment, your loyalty, your dedication to the community.

Needless to say, the GP training scheme gave you the opportunity to maximise your chances. You could do this by;

a) Adding to your qualifications. So at the end of your obstetrics stint, you could take the Diploma of the Royal College of Obstetricians and Gynaecologists (DRCOG). At the end of your paediatric job, you could take the Diploma in Child Health (DCH). And the crowning glory, on completion of your scheme, you could take the examination to become a Member of the Royal College of General Practitioners (MRCGP). Notwithstanding the formidable task of collecting these letters after your name, it had to be accomplished alongside your onerous house jobs, and in my case, trying to be a husband and father. Despite all this, it is something that almost all my colleagues were doing, so prospective interview panels would be faced with about a hundred almost identical applications, all ending with 'so please give me the job. Yours sincerely, Dr. John Smith, MBBS, DCH, DRCOG, MRCGP.'

b) You could use your three years to cosy up to the local practices, waiting for a vacancy to arise at the end. All very well, if you had decided to stay in the area in which you had undertaken your training. A good option, and many people did just that.

My training practice.

This consisted of a partnership of six doctors, practising out of a residential property, which was not designed to deliver 20th century medicine, although they were planning to move to a new purpose built super-duper building sometime during my tenure.

On my first day, they provided me with a very valuable experience. I was to spend the whole day sitting in the waiting room, pretending to be a patient, but actually undergoing the patient experience – the waiting, the frustration, the gripes, and the chat. Amazing what you hear in those situations – who likes which doctor, opinions and advice offered on the various complaints, local gossip, where to get your car fixed, and you'll never guess who is sleeping with....?! I made a point, in later years, of suggesting that medical students, who came to us as part of their training, underwent the same experience.

The senior partner was an exceedingly obese, bombastic individual who smoked cigars in the consulting room between patients. The other partners included;

-an elderly doctor, who was edging towards retirement and who just wanted to keep his head down for the next few years. He never disagreed with anyone, never contributed to meetings, never made a fuss. He had mastered the art of doing very little to expose himself to any form of risk. He would re-appoint almost all his patients at fortnightly intervals, just to check their blood pressure or keep an eye on their arthritis, depression, eczema or whatever. His entries in the medical record were miniscule, usually comprising the date, a blood pressure reading, and the single word 'Well'.

I remember one page of such a record which read;

February. 120/80. Well

March. 120/80. Well

April. 120/80. Well.

May. 120/80. Well.

June. 120/80. Well.

July. 120/80. Well.

August. 120/80. Well.

September. 120/80. Well.

October. Dead.

-a very Christian, very dedicated, constantly smiling doctor who thought he was the best doctor in the practice

-a short, thin, serious doctor who actually was the best doctor in the practice

-a slightly pompous upper-class chap with a penchant for silk wallpaper, even in his consulting room

-a huge, rugby playing Welshman, called Wyn, who took me under his wing, and who taught me most of what was important during my time there. He had an uncanny resemblance to Pavarotti, to the extent that, on one occasion on holiday, the convinced restaurant owner insisted on waiving the food and drink bill for the whole table, despite my friend's protestations. Quite how you can remain convinced when the person in question is saying 'Look now, boyo, I'm not him, you see.'

In the early days in the practice, you 'sit in' on consultations, and learn the art of general practice.

One day, a heavily tattooed female strode aggressively in to the consulting room, and, without saying a word, slammed a matchbox onto the desk. Wyn tentatively opened the box to reveal a piece of tissue paper, and several black dots.

'Crabs' she shouted, 'what am I going to do with those?'

Wyn looked at her, then at me, then closed the box.

'I suggest you poach them and serve them in a thermidor sauce.'

On another occasion, another red-faced aggressive individual (he did have calm patients also) burst into the room, pointed at Wyn and kicked off..

'You bastard, you absolute tosser...'

'Goodbye.' Said Wyn, without looking up from his notes.

'What the.....'

'Goodbye.'

'You can't just....'

'In two days, you will receive a letter removing you from the practice list. You can register elsewhere.'

'But...'

'Shut the door on your way out.'

'Just..'

'Door!'

The patient duly left. (Wyn is 6 feet two and 16 stones).

Seeing the look of protest on my face, he said 'Our job is difficult enough, we don't need to put up with that shit.'

I disagreed with him at the time, and forty years later, I still do. Angry patients are often frightened, confused, bewildered, or just plain angry. They might have had some bad news, been kept waiting an unreasonable amount of time, they might not know how to deal with their emotions, their illness, their medication. The least they can expect is to be heard. It is also likely that some of the anger and aggression would have been visited on the reception staff.

My strategy would be to say something like 'Hey, you sound really angry, sit down and tell me what's going on.' The problem would hopefully be revealed and dealt with. I would sometimes conclude the consultation by saying 'and if you had a go at the receptionist, it's not her fault, so perhaps you could say sorry on the way out.' They invariably did.

On a training course for reception staff, the issue of aggressive patients was raised. A maxim that proved extremely helpful was 'it is difficult to have an argument with someone who is agreeing with you.' So when a patient decided to have a go at the receptionist because they had been waiting half an hour to be seen, the response would be 'I fully understand. If *I'd* been waiting as long as you have, I'd be *really* cross.'

There were two outstanding features of my training practice.

Firstly, the characters described above disliked each other. They really did. They found it hard to be civil to each other, they did not socialise outside the practice, they grunted at each other as they passed in the corridor. But the absolute highlight was the fortnightly practice meeting. This was held in the evening, after surgery had finished, and starred the partners, the practice manager, the office manager, and of course, myself. These were very bad tempered affairs, with controversial agendas, and much backbiting. Chief amongst the contentious issues was the fact that the exceedingly obese senior partner had taken it upon himself to supervise the construction of the new surgery. This meant rearranging whole surgery sessions at short notice to go swanning around the half-built edifice for an afternoon, deciding on the light fittings and taps. Tempers flared, and it was not uncommon for a halt to be called in the proceedings whilst everyone filed out onto the pavement and paced up and down, muttering under their breath, to calm down sufficiently to allow the meeting to progress.

Secondly, these same characters were experts in 'The Red Book.'

The red book in question was actually called 'The Statement of Fees and Allowances.'

Remember the scandal about MPs expenses a few years ago? Outrageous claims being made for meals, interior design, hairdressers, duck houses in the moat on the country estate? 'Flipping' houses to maximise rent rebates? A national disgrace!

Ha! A bunch of amateurs. Absolute beginners.

The 'red book' set out what GPs were entitled to claim in order to be able to continue their noble profession, and what was 'allowable' when building new premises, or modifying existing premises.

Although it did not contain that many pages and sections, every word was pored over by obsessional GPs, avid to extract every penny from the government, which they viewed as their entitlement, after years of pay restraint and false promises. My practice had taken this activity to an art form.

For example, you could reasonably claim expenses for use of a car – this would include road tax, insurance, fuel, cleaning, servicing etc. But you could also claim a proportion of the expenses of a second car, as of course there was the possibility that your first car could malfunction in some way, creating the necessity for an emergency back-up vehicle.

You might occasionally ask patients to come to your home (never) for an out-of-hours consultation, so naturally, you would need to create the right environment to welcome such patients. A perfect garden creates a good impression, so claim for the gardener and the plants. Your hallway is the next point of entry, so claim for the decoration, the carpet, the cleaner, the Mr. Sheen polish.

Security is paramount, the burglar alarm essential, but you also need a dog, so claim for the dog food, the vet's bills, the disposable poo bags.

If you think this is ridiculous, move on to the regulations regarding the building of a new surgery. Permissible room sizes are specified, together with number of rooms, (you would obviously need one room per doctor, one room per nurse, a spare for locums and trainees, and one for training medical students), wall coverings, door handles, light fittings, cupboards, desks, chairs. In general, anything that was 'fixed' was easier to justify than anything that was 'moveable', so all desks and cupboards were built in, examination lamps were screwed to the wall, even chairs in reception were bolted to the floor.

I learned a lot. *This* 'red book' was more important than '*The thoughts of Chairman Mao*', though doubtless he would have approved.

Interviews

About six months from the end of my three year training programme, I nervously approached the process of applying for a post in general practice. As previously mentioned, I had chosen a good year. In 1985, there were, on average, one hundred applicants for every available general practice position. I had prepared an excellent CV, and I had had one hundred copies professionally printed. Every week, I scoured the pages of the BMJ, looking for suitable advertisements. We had already decided that, after three years in the West Midlands, we yearned to return to the south of England, so focussed our attention there.

The process began.

Slowly but surely the rejections started to arrive.

'Dear Doctor Hughes,

Thank you for the interest you have shown in our practice vacancy. We were overwhelmed by the response, and it has been a very difficult task to compile a shortlist. Unfortunately, on this occasion, we are unable to offer you an interview, but we feel sure that you will be successful in the near future.'

After about a dozen similar letters, I had my first interview, in Guildford.

I arrived far too early and found myself in a waiting area with two other candidates. I eyed them suspiciously, wondering which one of us was going to win the coveted prize.

'First time, is it?' asked the lanky pretender in the brown suit.

'Yes', I replied, slightly taken aback.

'They've already been through three this morning.'

His name was called and he left the room, glancing back as he did so.

'See you next week', he muttered.

He proved to be unerringly accurate in his prediction. As the interviews came and went, I became familiar with a few members of our cohort, to the extent we would even compare CVs to see where we were going wrong.

The weeks went by. At this point I was averaging an interview a week. I was unbelievably optimistic.

I went to one practice in Wiltshire, where the partners had struggled to produce a shortlist they could agree on, so they had decided to interview fifty candidates, yes *fifty*, over two days. I was somewhere in the middle of day two. I had driven for three hours, not even been offered a cup of tea, then shepherded into a room where I was faced with a very bored panel, asking boring questions.

'What is it that most interested you about our practice?'

I really had had enough, tired, thirsty, and appalled.

'At this moment in time, I really haven't got the faintest idea', I replied, 'I appear to be wasting my time and yours.' I got up and left.

They offered me the job. I turned it down. They contacted my trainer, asking me to reconsider. They loved my spirit and my honesty.

I told them that I would never consider working for a practice that did not offer a prospective partner a cup of tea.

Some practices asked for the wife or partner to come along to the interview. We drove to one such interview in Surrey. I met the partners in the afternoon, my heavily pregnant wife was shown around the practice and the local area. Very promising. In the evening, we were invited to the home of the senior partner. Having left home at lunchtime, we were by now completely famished. As we entered his lovely home, we were greeted by the lovely smell of food, a boeuf bourguignon, I fancied. His homely wife appeared and said, 'Dinner will be in fifteen minutes.'

'Righto, my dear.' He then proceeded to talk about the history of the practice and to show us the previous year's accounts, all very impressive.

The wife made another appearance. 'Five minutes', she said, impatiently.

We were salivating. The senior partner rounded up his deliberations.

'Come through' said his wife.

We all stood up.

'Good of you to come all this way' he said, shaking my hand, 'Safe journey.'

'Would you like to use the toilet before you go?' added his homely wife.

We drove to the nearest village, in a state of utter bewilderment, and had greasy fish and chips, before driving the three hours home.

A couple of months into the process, my wife said 'I just don't know how you cope with the rejections, and the letters, and the let-downs.'

'You have to believe in yourself' I say, brightly. 'When your ego is down to the dying embers, you have to throw another log on the fire.'

But we decide to revisit my CV, to see if there are any glaring errors or omissions. My mother-in-law suggests that I lie about my place of birth (Ireland), and shave off my beard, as I look like an IRA terrorist. Helpful.

Perhaps more dispiriting than the outright rejections were the occasions when you made it to the final two or three.

I'm down to the final two in a practice in leafy Surrey. This place has its own 'millionaires row' with pop stars, politicians, captains of industry. They show me the accounts, including the mind-blowing income from private practice. I meet the charming junior partner, who tells me that he has just bought a tiny two-bedroom house for £83,000. (This is 1985, remember). Everything is going swimmingly. The next week, I get *the letter*. A few months later, at a conference, I happen to meet the successful candidate, lovely chap. He offers his commiserations, and then adds 'I hate to tell you this, but you were the preferred candidate.

However the senior partner overruled the others on the grounds that your Northern accent might grate with some of the private patients.'

Ee bah gum, there's nowt so queer as folk. Of course, he has a point. There I am, ministering to Lord Hawdihaw, when I suddenly burst in to a rousing chorus of 'On Ilkley moor b'aht 'at', pull my cloth cap on and do a clog dance in the bedroom. Unseemly.

I'm down to the last two in a small practice in Bournemouth. Modern, progressive, young partners, great premises, good ideas.

I really want this one. I really do.

It is on a Saturday morning when *the letter* arrives. Handwritten, kind, *difficult decision, sure you'll find a position soon.* My wife arrives in the kitchen to find me weeping uncontrollably. She tells me to go back to bed. A short while later, she brings me up a cup of tea, and a plate on which she has placed some cardboard cut-outs of logs. 'Throw another log on that fire', she gently says.

July 1985. A five man practice on the south coast. Nice partners, nice views, a cramped, converted, 19th century seaside villa, now masquerading as a doctor's surgery, and serving a population of 10,000.

I'm down to the last two.

One evening, I get a phone call from the senior partner.

'We would be delighted if you would accept our offer of a partnership, and join us in September.'

There is much rejoicing in the Hughes household that evening. We tell our families, all our friends, our neighbours, anyone who will listen, and we do some serious damage to a bottle of Glenfiddich we have been saving for just such an occasion.

Everyone is happy for us. Except my mother.

"Well, you couldn't have moved much further away from me if you tried.' (she lives in Lancashire).

I choose not to mention the two failed applications to Jersey.

Of course, I feel desperately sad for the other guy. I needn't have worried. Within weeks of the original advertisement, another partner in the same practice decides to up sticks and head off to a career on medical politics. So the practice offers the post to him.

The new practice

I am a GP.

I have my own consulting room, with my name on the door.

I have a brass plate on the wall outside the surgery.

And I have truly fallen on my feet.

My new practice is a friendly five person practice in a seaside town. Some of the consulting rooms have a sea view. As the junior partner, mine does not, but I only have to go into the coffee room to enjoy sweeping views of the English Channel.

Each partner works four full days and has a day off, which is rostered every two years for fairness. There is a sensible on-call evening rota, shared with another practice in town, meaning that you work half a weekend every five weeks. There is a strong emphasis on quality of life and co-operative working.

Apart from myself, there is the senior partner, Len, a rotund avuncular Welshman, who is fond of sailing and whisky. There are two married female partners with families, and James, who joined the practice at the same time as me. James is the same age as me, married, enthusiastic, and it soon becomes obvious that we share common goals for the practice, and indeed, for life. Over the next thirty-odd years, he is to become not only my partner in the practice, but my best friend, next-door neighbour, business partner, fellow holidaymaker, and drinking buddy.

Fortunate indeed.

In the first week, Len suggests I join him on an on-call evening to 'familiarise myself with the practice area'. We set off to respond not only to requests for home visits, but also to 'pop in' on some of his favourite patients. Each visit seems to follow a startlingly similar path. 'Evening, Len, time for a small one?' He introduces me as the 'new boy' and we all have a whisky. Several visits later, I am feeling a bit off-kilter, but Len is still in his element. 'Aren't you worried about drinking and driving?' I nervously propose. 'All the cops know my car' is his astonishingly frank reply. At the end of the evening I fell into bed. The next morning, my wife complained bitterly about my snoring. 'Exhaustion' I explained, shame-faced.

The cops do know his car. I had overlooked the fact that, in addition to the routine of normal GP work, our practice was 'on-call' for the local police station. We could be called upon to take blood samples from drunk drivers, certify death in murders, section mentally ill offenders, and so on. One Friday evening, a few weeks into my new role, I had been relaxing after a busy week, still celebrating my good fortune, and ready for bed after two or three decent whiskies. The phone went. 'Sorry to bother you, doctor, PC Sumner here, we have a chap at the station, picked up driving erratically, just needs a blood alcohol doing.' I had entirely forgotten that I was on the rota that night. A quick cup of coffee and some peppermints later, I turned up at the station. Hoping that my aim would be true, I obtained the necessary sample and was about to make a quick escape when the duty officer said 'we have another one coming in, doc, might as well nip down the canteen and get yourself a coffee.' A young PC offered to show me the way and proceeded to sit opposite me over the disgusting coffee. I was praying that he wouldn't smell my breath, or notice the slightly blood shot eyes. I eventually made it home safely.

The following Monday, I confess my sins to Len. 'Don't worry about it' he says, 'but next time, tell them you've had a few, and ask them to send a car for you. That's what I always do.'

ECT – a shocking experience

Electroconvulsive therapy (ECT) is a procedure, done under general anaesthesia, which is used to treat severe depression and other major psychiatric illnesses. It consists of passing an electric current through the brain, triggering a seizure. The theory behind this procedure is that the electrical stimulus causes the release of certain chemicals in the brain, which might alleviate the symptoms of severe depression or mania, which has proved resistant to other forms of therapy. Side effects of ECT can include confusion, memory loss (which can persist for months), and physical effects such as headache and muscle pain. Naturally, therefore, it is a treatment option reserved for the most serious cases.

In case this description brings to mind images from Hammer House of Horror films, where the mad scientist sends a huge surge of buzzing electricity into the brain of the monster / creature / zombie, and the meter registers 10,000 Volts (marked DANGER!! In red), well, let me put your mind at ease. Sort of.

My internet sources, mostly written for patients, tell me that;

-you will have a full physical assessment prior to the procedure

-you will have an intravenous line inserted

-you will be given an anaesthetic and a muscle relaxant

-monitors will check your brain, heart, blood pressure and oxygen levels

-after the procedure, you will be taken to a recovery area, where you will be monitored for potential problems.

Happier now?

Well, perhaps I am suffering from confusion and memory loss...

It is 1984 (the year, not the book), and I have been a junior psychiatric doctor for three weeks. At the day hospital, the ward sister announces that it is the ECT session today. An anaesthetist turns up, and the first patient arrives on the trolley. I seem to remember some sort of straps or restraints being involved. Sister brings in the ECT machine, which looks pre-war, and what looks like a set of cheap headphones. The anaesthetist gives the patient a slug of something, sister hands me the electrodes, I put them in the required location, turn up the dial as instructed and click the switch. A vigorous and prolonged convulsion occurs. This whole performance is repeated three or four times on different patients, the anaesthetist waves cheery-bye, and we are left with a roomful of individuals at different stages of the recovery process. ECG monitor? No. EEG monitor? You must be joking. Oxygen monitor? They weren't in use then. Blood pressure monitor? Nope. The only thing connected to the poor unsuspecting patient was the national grid, well, a modified version of it.

Later in my career, as a junior anaesthetist, I was ordained to travel, once a month, to a remote mental hospital resembling something out of an Agatha Christie novel, and give the knock-out juice to up to six patients, who, after the ECT, would be lined up in a small recovery area supervised by one nurse.

I know that there are many papers in learned journals purporting to show the benefits of ECT, but, from my experience, it never seemed to make any positive difference, and I still consider it to be medieval and barbaric. You will, point out, I hope, that my sample of participants is too small to be of statistical significance, and this is indeed so, but I don't think that even the most optimistic supporter would echo the brio of those laughable hair commercials;

'ECT – because you're worth it!' (71% of 95 users agree.)

Farmers

They are a breed apart.

Our practice had, on its northern boundary, a number of small farms, mainly livestock. We rarely visited them, so at times they were difficult to find. Directions such as 'We're not hard to find, it's the Old Farm on Old Farm Lane' were less than helpful. Pre sat-nav, we had to rely on broken gates, knarled trees and milk churn stands as waymarkers.

A typical visit would go something like this. I would drive my entirely unsuitable family saloon up a rutted track full of mud, puddles and animal excrement, to arrive in front of a solid stone built house. The spacious yard would be littered with rusting agricultural machinery. A snarling, muscular, mythical beast called Cerberus or Satan would hurl itself repeatedly at the car, testing the integrity of a chain, which, in a previous life, would have ended in a ship's anchor.

'Don't mind him, doc, he's harmless.'

 The farmer's wife, dressed in a headscarf, Barbour jacket, corduroy trousers and sturdy wellies, would then lead me down stone-flagged hallways in to a huge kitchen, the centrepiece of which would be a pine table the size of my front garden, on which would be piled old newspapers, bank statements, tin boxes and assorted bits and bridles. Often, there would be a box of shotgun cartridges for good measure. Farmer Giles would be sitting on an ancient rocking chair in front of a roaring fire. You might be tempted to think that this is some sort of rustic idyll conjured up out of my imagination, based on sketches from the *Two Ronnies*, but I assure you that this was the backdrop against which many visits were set.

One visit involved the farmer's wife herself. She greeted me cheerily, waving a bandaged hand. 'Sorry I couldn't come down to the surgery, can't drive the Land Rover one-handed.'

A brief inspection revealed an ancient, loosely applied bandage, held together with Sellotape. Once removed, I was confronted with a badly infected wound to the right hand, with cellulitis spreading up the forearm.

'One of the animals got a bit frisky last week, damn thing bit me. I tried bathing it in warm vinegar, but it's starting to smart a bit now.' The woman had a life threatening infection, bordering on septicaemia. She required urgent admission and intravenous antibiotics. God knows what pain she endured soaking an open wound in malt vinegar.

On another occasion, it was the farmer who had prompted the call. 'Been getting a bit short of breath, doc.' The reason was obvious. He couldn't breathe because his abdomen was filled with twenty or thirty litres of fluid, pushing up on his diaphragm and compressing his lungs. He was also a deep shade of orange. I took his wife aside and delivered the bad news.

'I am afraid he has advanced cancer of the liver.'

'Thought as much.' She nodded knowingly.

'Why didn't he come to see me earlier?'

'Well, you know what he's like, stubborn bastard.'

I did not know what he was like. I had never seen him before. Neither had anyone else from the medical profession. His GP notes did not contain a single entry for the previous forty years.

I admitted him to hospital where he died two days later.

On other occasions, you might catch sight of a shadowy figure lurking in one of the barns. 'That's just Jed, my youngest. He's a bit slow, keeps himself to himself.' In other words 'He has an undiagnosed mental illness, of which social services and the mental health services are completely unaware, but whilst he is here under our protection, he remains completely harmless'. Put him in a red check shirt and braces, and he would not be out of place in *Deliverance*, let alone a south coast rural community.

And all of the above characters would be the very same people who would need my signature every so often to confirm that they were eligible to renew their shotgun licence.

Treehugging

In 1990s general practice, the trend was *Reflective Practice*. I suppose these days we would call it *Mindfulness* or *Hygge*, or some such passing phrase. A two-day course was advertised, and, as we were both members of the prestigious Royal College of General Practitioners, it was decided that both James and myself would go.

We arrived at some woodland retreat in the Cotswolds, and found ourselves in a large meeting room with about thirty reflective GPs from the region. Our guides for the next two days were a large woman with spiky hair, who was wearing a shapeless smock and Albanian shepherd's boots, and an overly enthusiastic bearded man wearing brown corduroy trousers and 'Cornish pasty' shoes. I guess at this point I should say 'spoiler alert'.

The spiky haired woman opened the proceedings.

'We do not want this to be a directive encounter, so instead of putting you into groups, we would like you to move towards a space in the room where you feel comfortable.'

We all looked at each other, and shuffled in a less-than-comfortable manner into six, roughly evenly-sized groups.

We were then advised to move to our 'break-out' rooms, where we would find a flipchart and pens, and we would discuss topics such as 'what makes a good doctor?' or 'is change challenging?'

After the allotted time, we reassembled, and fed back our thoughts to the whole group. When it came to our turn, we turned to our self-appointed leader, who was now sitting at the back of the room, leaning back on his chair, with his feet on the back of the chair in front, revealing a pair of alarmingly red socks.

'There was a flipchart in our room' he said 'but it didn't want to join our group, so we have nothing to report.'

There was a short silence.

'That's absolutely fine' said the spiky one.

'Fine' echoed the corduroy pants.

It was not fine.

In the afternoon, we had a session on *conflict*.

'I'm going to make a statement to the group. I'd like you to consider it, then offer a response. Here is the statement….'I think this course is going really well.'

There was a reflective pause. Then Red Socks piped up.

'What course are *you* on?'

We made it, rather painfully, through the rest of the leaden day, before rushing to the nearest pub in the evening. There was a sort of an 'emperor's new clothes' atmosphere, until one plucky chap said 'Is it just me, or is this a load of bollocks?' We all heartily agreed, and relaxed over a few drinks.

The next morning, we waded through more sessions. Then we all promised to explore *patient empowerment*, to introduce *shared decision making* into our consultations, and to sit cross-legged every morning and chant 'OM' to the goddess of dawn. We left at lunchtime, and went back to the real world.

Gifts

Gifts. From patients. Always a tricky one, that.

The General Medical Council in its *Good practice Guidelines* states;

You must not ask for or accept – from patients, colleagues or others – any inducement, gift or hospitality that may affect or be seen to affect the way you prescribe for, treat or refer patients or commission services for patients. You must not offer these inducements.

It makes sense if you think about it. Whilst it might seem churlish, hurtful even, to refuse a small 'thank you' from a grateful patient, it has a different perspective when the gift is more substantial. Is the doctor going to be compromised in future dealings with the patient? Is the patient going to start making unreasonable requests, for the doctor's time, for prescriptions, for preferential treatment, all on the basis of 'that nice present I gave you.'?

There was a famous, indeed infamous, GP in the 1950s called Bodkin Adams. He worked in Eastbourne, and he was a suspected serial killer. Between 1946 and 1956, more than 160 of his patients died in suspicious circumstances. Of these, more than 130 had left him money or items in their wills. He was actually tried for murder in 1957, and acquitted. One of his patients, Alice Morrell, died in 1949, leaving him a small amount of money, and some cutlery. Oh, and a Rolls Royce. Another patient, Gertrude Hullett, died in 1956. She left him several valuable items in her will. Oh, and a Rolls Royce. He was eventually struck off the Medical Register for forging prescriptions – but later reinstated! At the time of his death, aged 83, his fortune was over £400,000. He had been receiving legacies until his death.

I have never been particularly fortunate in the gift stakes, so compromising my professional integrity has never been a major worry. That Bentley I forgot to mention, the gold Rolex I use to check whether I am running to time...

Even within my own narrow ambit, there have been others more fortunate than myself. One local GP inherited a farm. A farm, for God's sake! Another was left a vintage car. And someone with close ties to the BMA is fond of pointing out in his lectures, that he was left a small fortune in a will just because he looked after a patient's parrot whilst she was in hospital.

At a dinner party hosted by a good friend and colleague, post-prandial refreshment was being offered. 'What do you fancy?' he asked and opened a large wooden drinks cabinet to reveal an impressive range of single malt whiskies, fine ports, and five star brandies. 'Good Lord!' I exclaimed, 'you've certainly pushed the boat out!'

'All gifts, dear boy, mostly at Christmas.' He went on to explain that it had been his custom, as the festive season drew close, to wrap a whisky-shaped bottle in Christmas paper, and leave it on a shelf behind his desk, in the direct eye line of the incoming patient. 'That's a good idea' they would think, and lo and behold, another similar package arrives and is duly deposited in the drinks cabinet.

'I'll try that,' I thought. It generated some sort of response, but not of the Macallan variety. Think Blue Nun or the dreaded Harvey's Bristol Cream. It's not that there is anything wrong with Harvey's Bristol Cream. Well there is actually, it is awful stuff. Thankfully, I was able to strike a deal with our local shop – I gave them the Harvey's, they gave me an equivalent amount of red wine.

A few years ago, I was looking after a charming retired antiques dealer, who had terminal lung cancer. I would drop in to see him at home, to discuss his condition, his pain control, his last wishes. On such visits, he would often show me items from his personal collection. He had excellent taste. When he died, his widow came to see me to thank me for my care and compassion. 'Charles was very fond of you. He told me 'When I've gone, make sure you get the doctor a decent case of wine.' My heart quickened at the thought. Some Chateauneuf – du –Pape, perhaps. No, some decent Sauternes. Wait, he had *exceptional* taste. Could it be Chateau Lafite, surely not?

'I'm not well versed in these matters,' she said 'so I have arranged for something to be delivered.'

A week later, an impressive box from a well-known vintner's arrived at the surgery. It contained six bottles of Harvey's Bristol Cream.

Things in places they shouldn't oughta be

I cannot possibly hope to compete with the myriad medical tales about all sorts of things in all sorts of places.

I suspect that most are possibly untrue, or have been subject to extreme embellishment in the telling and re-telling.

So, for the record, I have never had to treat anyone with an injury to the penis caused by a vacuum cleaner. (Although there is an excellent article on the subject, reported in the extremely serious *British Medical Journal*, which even gives advice on the models and attachments to be avoided.)

And I have never had to assess the damage to the nethers caused by accidentally sitting on a sink plunger whilst cleaning the bathroom in the nude.

But I *did* work in the same hospital where twenty metres of copper wire were extracted (through the penis) from the bladder of an post office engineer. His explanation? 'Well, it has never got stuck before.' Candid, and sensible. Much better to admit that you have an interesting hobby, than to face the withering stare that expresses thinly disguised disbelief and amusement from a seasoned professional, as you spin the most improbable of fairy stories.

One such encounter, in my general practice, involved a married man in his fifties whose discomfort, as he sat before me in the surgery, turned out to be physical as well as emotional. For reasons best known to himself, he had inserted a whole, peeled cucumber into his rectum. It had inconveniently snapped in half, leaving him holding in his hand what, in different circumstances, would have the makings of a nice salad. What to do about the other half? I told him that attempts to remove it would be fruitless (no pun intended), that it was vegetable matter, would quickly degrade and be passed in the usual way. Maybe don't peel it next time? (more stability).

I was also asked to visit an elderly man in his home, who was complaining of 'waterworks problems'. I started to examine him, and was surprised to find that inside his underpants, his entire genitalia were shrouded in a waxy Warburton's bread wrapper. Disguising my surprise, I carefully removed it to reveal wads of toilet paper. When these were discarded, I was startled to see what looked like a bit of metal protruding from the 'eye' of his penis. It was indeed a three inch long brass screw, which he deftly withdrew. 'It helps to stop the water leaking out', he explained, as if it was a most reasonable solution. 'Not very hygienic', I offered. 'I change it every day!' he proclaimed indignantly. The poor man had advanced prostate problems, thankfully not malignant, and easily remedied by a surgical procedure. I don't know if, once cured, he changed from Warburton's, although it does make very nice toast.

During my time on the geriatric ward, I received a call from a local GP, requesting the admission of an elderly lady with a complex mix of social, psychiatric and physical problems. The social element comprised severe self-neglect, to the extent that it was no longer safe for her to live independently. The psychiatric problem was increasing dementia. The medical problem was recurring genital and urinary tract infections, a contributory factor seeming to be her habit of putting potatoes in her vagina. At the end of my shift, the patient had still not arrived, so I handed the problem over to a new doctor, who gave the impression of having just stepped off the plane from Mumbai. His name was Dr. Mistry. Dr. A. Mistry. Really. I went through the details of the expected admission. When I came to the bit about the potatoes, his eyes widened, and his head bobbled about vigorously.

'Oh, no, no, no. I am not understanding this' he pleaded. He looked like he was about to cry.

I went through the details once more.

'No, no, no, no. This is not making any sense to me. The head bobbled so much, I feared it might lead to a concussion.

At this point, I should have taken the time to explain the complex interrelationship between social factors, the ageing process, and the presence of co-morbidities in the mental and physical health spectrum of the human condition.

It was now 6 p.m.. I had been on duty for 34 hours. There was a glass of red wine waiting for me at home. I left the ward, with these words of advice.

'Look, mate, if she clears her plate at supper, just make sure it's all in her stomach, OK?'

Other things in other places...

A post mortem report on one of my elderly patients, who had died following a fall in a nursing home, revealed the incidental finding of a *trichobezoar* in her stomach. This is a large mass of hair, akin to the fur balls that cats often develop. It is usually the result of biting the ends of the hair over prolonged periods of time. Anyway, it had sat happily in her stomach, possibly for decades, acquiring a degree of calcification, and had not apparently done her any harm.

And I will be forever indebted to the mother who brought her small child to see me, concerned that he had swallowed a five pence piece. It gave me the opportunity, after many years in practice, to use that famous music hall riposte – 'Ring me if there's any change.'

Rogues and villains

Every person living in Great Britain and Northern Ireland has the right to be registered with a general practitioner. Even bad people. In a practice of 10,000 individuals you would expect your fair share of alcoholics, drug abusers, sociopaths, paedophiles – the sort of people that society might designate as 'bad people' – but to us they are patients, people in need of our help, treatment possibly.

Then there are the rogues and villains – people who are 'just the wrong side of the law', but likeable perhaps. In this motley crew, there are 'the fixers' – people who can get you things –a brace of pheasants, duty free cigarettes and booze, line-caught sea bass. Of course, we have to maintain a professional, detached attitude to such offerings, but apparently, supermarket sea bass comes a poor second. Gently fried in butter with a lemon sauce, served with some mashed potatoes and greens. Delicious, so I'm told.

Then there are the 'tradesmen' – shifty characters operating for cash, who can fit a kitchen, repair your roof, do an extension. Always ready to drop their business card on the desk at the end of a consultation. And why not? You are hardly likely to do a duff job on the plastering, knowing that the 'customer' might have your balls in his hand at some point in the future – medically speaking, of course.

One of my favourites was a big, beefy guy who had worked in the prisons, then worked in 'security', and now running a small business. Brawny, tattooed, scar-faced. He drove a Subaru, or some other sort of ridiculous, testosterone fuelled excuse of a car. (I am always tempted to ask such individuals how Sue Barrow is doing,) and most consultations featured his latest exploits, whether it was outrunning the police when he was speeding, drinking phenomenal amounts of Newcastle Brown and then driving home, or sorting out some loudmouth lads in the early hours, on his way back from the pub. All this with a pinch of salt, but he was not the sort of person you would want to cross. One day he arrived for his appointment, and informed me that some 'arsehole' was giving the receptionists a hard time downstairs, and did I want him to go and sort him out? It was very tempting. Unfortunately, his lifestyle had contributed to the development of type 2 diabetes, which was why I had regular consultations with him. Obese, appalling diet, hypertensive, smoker, heavy drinker, stressed, raised cholesterol, he posed quite a challenge. I repeatedly outlined his risks, and the myriad ways in which I could help him to reduce them. He was having none of it. He had a sort of death wish, and was not prepared to compromise his way of living for a complication-free existence. Ultimately, the complications started to arrive in the form of liver disease, kidney disease, and angina. At this point, he 'saw the light' and made strenuous efforts to reform. He had modest success, and whilst it may have increased his life expectancy, I am ashamed to admit that he became a less interesting character.

Real undesirables were not hard to find. One of the worst was Rick, a proper scumbag (not a medical diagnosis, but accurate nevertheless). He was a convicted criminal, thief, burglar, he had done time for a bit of GBH, and he had a drug habit. This was mostly benzodiazepines, so he was always on the make for some diazepam (Valium), for 'his nerves'. One Friday evening, he confronted me in the surgery, demanding more supplies. I politely refused his request, whereupon he grabbed my tie and started to 'adjust' it in an upward direction. I reconsidered his very reasonable request.

A few months later, Rick was found dead in a hovel of a flat, having had a stroke. **Don't mess with me**. I stopped wearing ties in the surgery from that day on, citing a recent article in the BMJ on infection control that suggested the GPs never cleaned their germ-ridden ties (true).

Another incident concerned a rather immature, but violent young man, who had unrealistic expectations about the sort of care he should be receiving for his problems, and about the level of benefits he was entitled to. One day, I pointed all this out to him. He left the surgery in a rage, only to return a couple of hours later, fuelled by lager. He stormed into my room, interrupting a consultation, shouted and swore at me, called me various names, berating me for my attitude towards him. 'I'm seeing a patient at the moment' I said, more calmly than I felt 'make an appointment if you wish to discuss this further.' He glared around, shouted 'You are dead', slammed the door and left. Unfortunately, the upper door of the surgery was locked, so he had to make his way downstairs, meekly saying 'excuse me' to the waiting patients, and make an ignominious exit.

A few months later, his lifeless body was washed up on a beach 20 miles away. Like I said, **don't mess with me.**

Murder, suicide, and coroners

In the very first week in my new practice there was a double murder in the town. One of my partners was called out to confirm the deaths. This was a great shock to me, as I had told my friends and family that I was moving to one of the safest places in the UK. It proved to be a one-off (or more correctly, a two-off), as there was only one more murder in my patch in the next thirty years.

Suicide, on the other hand, is much more common. There are still 4500 suicides in this country per year, although numbers are falling. In 2018, a suicide prevention minister was appointed by Theresa May as part of the government's commitment to tackling mental health issues. I remain unconvinced that the vast majority of suicides are preventable. Before I get roundly criticised by the mental health lobbyists, let me quickly say that my opinions are shaped by my own personal experiences. Most 'successful' suicides that occurred over my career were unpredictable, sudden and shocking. Suicide is very distressing for the friends and family, more so perhaps than death due to natural causes, because of its suddenness and the many unanswered questions. Let us not forget also the impact on the health care professionals involved in the case. Every one of the suicides that occurred in our practice led to intensive soul searching and scrutiny of the medical record, to see if anything was missed – any vital clue which might have saved a life. It was rare to find any glaring faults or omissions, whilst many patients were known to the mental health services, there was seldom any crucial indicator that a life was to be taken. One of my colleagues suffered a long period of low mood following one of these cases, with a good degree of self-blame, although independent assessment of the case proved that there were no opportunities to change the course of events.

Parasuicide is a term which is often applied to 'failed' suicide attempts. These are very common indeed, and are often classified as 'calls for help' – the person involved not fully intending to take their life. This could be a non-fatal overdose of medication, a slash on the wrist, a threat to jump in front of a train. These failed attempts are generally thought to be a positive indicator of future success, and it is indeed these individuals where suicide prevention measures need to be maximally applied. Interestingly, about 95% of suicide attempts end in survival. Also, only about 15 – 30% of suicide victims leave a note. Those that do are less likely to have a history of psychiatric illness.

Anyway, as I said, most of the cases I encountered were completely unpredictable. With one exception. This concerned a man who I met as a GP trainee in the West Midlands. He was in his late fifties, an accountant who had taken early retirement. All was going well in his life, but over the course of a few weeks, he developed a profound and debilitating depression. He failed to respond to a variety of antidepressants, was referred to a psychiatrist, and was also seen by a psychologist. I can hardly recall any other patient who was immersed in dread, hopelessness and misery. He attempted suicide by taking tablets, but his wife had returned home early and caught him in the act. Judging from the pills he had in front of him, he would have been undoubtedly successful. From then on, his wife locked all pills and medicines out of his way. On another occasion, his wife stopped him, and unbelievably *searched* him, just as he was going out for a walk. He had secreted a ten inch chef's knife in his clothing. His wife, understandably, was desperate, and I had several consultations with her to try to decide a way forward.

She telephoned me in the early hours one morning, to say that she had found her husband, dead, in the kitchen. He had consumed a household poison, and was indeed dead. He had apparently achieved his goal.

Due to the nature of the death, it became a coroner's case. I was summonsed to attend. My first time before the coroner, and an experience I would not rush to repeat. I was made to feel, throughout the procedure, as though I had poured the poison directly down the unfortunate man's throat. The coroner's questions were probing, intrusive, accusatory almost. I was anxious, I was sweating profusely as the onslaught continued.

'Are you telling me, doctor, that this man was able to consume such a large volume of poison without vomiting?'

'Yes, sir.'

'How much exactly do you think he imbibed?'

'Well, about five hundred millilitres, sir.'

'How can you be sure that the bottle was full to start with?'

'Because his wife told me it was.'

'How much was left in the bottle?'

'I don't know, about 200ml?'

Consults his notes.

'The police record says it was 300ml.'

I didn't know what to say to that. I was eventually dismissed, expecting to be clapped in irons and taken away.

The pathologist was next up, and was able to report that the deceased had indeed died of ingestion of poison. This poor man had poisoned his nervous system to the point that his brain cells ceased to function. I would not have thought it was possible. Neither, presumably, did the coroner. Coroners are appointed by the crown, and answer only to the crown. Scary. Especially when you are standing in front of one of them, a young, terrified, apprentice GP.

Break-ins and fires

I arrive early one morning to be greeted by a police car parked outside the surgery. I identify myself, and am informed that the cleaners arrived to find a crime scene. The rear window of the building had been forced, and attempts had been made to break into the controlled drugs cupboard. Some random damage elsewhere, nothing serious. The officer showed me the point of entry. 'Any chance of catching those responsible?' I half-heartedly asked. 'More than a fighting chance' he replied. He then indicated the window in question, where the fingerprint chaps had been doing their best. A perfect set of full hand and fingerprints emerged, where the Mastermind had planted both ungloved hands on the sash window to push it up. An arrest swiftly followed.

On another occasion, I arrived to a scene of devastation. In the treatment room, cupboards and drawers were left open, contents strewn over the floor, needles, tubing, and ampoules lying amongst bandages and swabs. 'Looks like another break-in', my razor-sharp intellect determined.

At that point, Peter, a locum doctor who had been working with us for a month, arrived. 'Er, that was me' he announced, embarrassed. The poor man had been called out, in the night, to a patient suffering a severe asthmatic attack. Not having all the necessary drugs and kit in his car, he made an emergency dash to the surgery, found everything he needed, and rushed off to save a life. Busy night, no time to return to clear things up. Forgiven.

In 1990, we had gone on a family skiing holiday, accompanied by James. In the middle of the week, he dutifully phoned his non-skiing wife, to update her on his remarkable black run feats, the excellent conditions, the hilarious apres-ski events. 'All OK at home?' he remembered to ask, eventually. 'The surgery burned down' was the monotone reply.

The practice, at that time occupied the lower two floors of a three storey Victorian building. The upper floor was home to a rather eccentric individual named Derek, who lived quietly and harmoniously, with his cat for company. On the evening in question, he had popped out for a drink, and as it was winter, he had left his moggy nestled on a folded, aged electric blanket to keep it warm. The fire investigation officer informed us that it might have been faulty wiring, coupled with feline urine that caused a short circuit, that led to the conflagration. The prompt response of the fire services rapidly extinguished the blaze, limiting the structural damage, but 100,000 gallons of water certainly fucks up your computers, your newly renovated consulting rooms, carpets, seating, lighting, ceilings. Thankfully, the paper medical records of 10,000 patients were unaffected, as they were in a different part of the building.

Amongst the embers of the upper storey flat, they recovered the charred remains of the cat. Smoky. Not a post-mortem diagnosis. His name.

The fire made the front pages of the local press. The report helpfully include the statement that 'at the time of the fire, Dr Hughes was in France on a family skiing holiday.' Helpful, in that it secured for me a pretty unassailable alibi in the event that I was a suspected arsonist. Helpful, also, if you were a burglar, guaranteed a trouble free visit to my unoccupied family home.

The pharmaceutical industry

When I was a junior hospital doctor, my contact with representatives of the pharmaceutical industry (henceforth 'reps') was very limited. Every so often, there would be what was known as a 'drug lunch' in the doctor's mess. This usually involved a rep laying on a buffet, some senior doctor giving a short talk about a medical matter, and a short presentation from the rep about a new wonder drug. We would turn up, wolf down a few sandwiches, listen to the talks, and then leave with pockets stuffed with pens and post-it notes. As doctors with very limited prescribing flexibility, we were not interested in the reps, similarly we were just not their target audience.

How things changed in general practice. Reps clamoured to see us, there were numerous inducements to prescribe their drugs, we were gods. Some practices banned reps completely, others welcomed them with open arms. We took the view that they were a necessary evil, and offered them proper appointments, rather than asking then to sit and wait for long periods until you could deign to see them after a full surgery. They always brought cakes for the girls on reception, which at least guaranteed them a chance of being seen. But cakes were just the thin end of the wedge. The whole practice, spouses included, would often be taken to dinner at the best restaurants in town, drinks included. This was technically against the rules, as spouses should not have been paid for, but the reps would get round it by saying 'well your wife is a nurse, so that's OK' (even if she wasn't).

Had we chosen to do so, we could have gone out to dinner with a different rep two or three times a week. And not just dinner – I would sometimes be taken out for lunch, with wine on offer, before returning to do afternoon surgery. Unthinkable in later years.

It did not stop there. No sensible doctor ever paid for a stethoscope, pen torch, tuning fork, tongue depressors (for saying 'Aaaah), otoscope (for looking in ears), medical books, or anything else for that matter. 'We need a new nebuliser (for asthma treatment).' No problem. You might accept that medical items were acceptable gifts, but we also had road maps, flashlights, mugs, toolkits, Swiss knives, mouse mats, car blankets. My children used to complain that everything in their Christmas stocking had a drug name on it. Well, apart from the satsuma.

If we needed to go to a medical conference, that could be arranged. In fact, most medical education was organised and sponsored by the industry. I even went on an all-expenses paid trip to a town in Germany 'to see the production facility' of a major pharmaceutical giant. We did see the facility, but we also had a trip up the Rhine, went to a beer Keller, and even a casino. Necessary medical education?

Then things changed, and rightly so. Pharmaceutical companies started to spy on each other, and report breaches of the Industry Code. No more meetings in lavish hotels, no more conferences on golf courses, no more foreign junkets. Then, no gifts with a value of greater than £6, then no gifts. Then no pens, no post-it notes. All income from the industry, such as lecture fees, to be properly documented, and declared. The companies themselves would alert you to the details they had been obliged to pass on to the taxman.

Having been a considerable beneficiary of the largesse of the drugs industry, I have to agree that these changes were long overdue, and absolutely necessary. There is no earthly way you can say, hand on heart, that prescribing patterns were not influenced by these blatant bribes. 'Shall I prescribe drug A, or drug B?' The one whose rep took me to Germany, perhaps.

A bit on the side

General practice is an immensely rewarding and fulfilling career. Every day is full of variety, working conditions are pleasant, remuneration is good, and you can look forward to a generous pension (correct at the time of writing). But you have to realise that most GPs become partners in the practice at the age of 28 or so, and therefore face the prospect of doing the same thing, in the same place, with the same people for the next 37 years (unless you retire early, as everyone seems to do at the present time).

Not surprising then, that many GPs look for something else to occupy their time. This may take the form of specialist work, research, work for government departments, politics, or something entirely different such as writing fiction, being a stand-up comedian, or a television personality. In most cases, this alternative activity runs in parallel with their general practice career, in some cases, it entirely supplants it. Having 'a bit on the side' stimulates creativity, it can be intellectually satisfying, it can even provide additional income for school fees, exotic holidays, second homes, or sailing (an appalling waste of time and money).

Part 1

My first 'bit on the side' happened whilst I was still in training. It came in the form of locum out-of-hours work in the evening. This was common practice, but was heavily frowned upon. The need or opportunity arose because, at the time, all GPs had to be on-call for their own patients after the practice was closed for the night. The occasional GP would prefer to sit at home with a nice whisky or two, instead of dashing out to see a child with a tummy ache or a wheezing asthmatic. The way it worked was this; I would be paid a retainer for the night. On top of this, I would get a fee for each visit I undertook. But the real money was for the 'night visit'. At the time, any visit requested and executed between the hours of 11 p.m. and 7 a.m. attracted a jolly nice fee – about £11 in the 1980s. Naturally, therefore, as a penniless junior doctor, every single call received between these hours clearly deserved a visit.

71

'I've got a bit of a cough.'

'I'll be straight out.'

'No need to bother yourself, doctor, I'm sure it will wait until the morning.'

'Could be something serious, better to check.'

Medication queries, itch rashes, earache – all desperately urgent medical emergencies. But there was a system of checks and balances – random patients were sent a questionnaire by the authorities asking whether the GP had *actually* visited, and *what time* the call was made. There was a sneaky way round this. If a patient called at 10.50 p.m. (as they infuriatingly did), you would say, 'Take some paracetamol, and if it's no better in an hour, call me back.' Multiple claims were thus generated, and it was no skin off the nose of the claiming GP, as he submitted the forms I had signed, and was paid by the authorities. The patients in their turn thought they were getting a fantastic service, as the enthusiastic young doctor never failed to visit.

Part 2

A few years after I joined the practice, a colleague asked if I would be interested in doing some work for the Benefits Agency. There was a shortage of doctors willing to undertake the work, and the pay was reasonably good. A brief interview, followed by some perfunctory training, then I was given a large manual to read, and I became a Benefits Assessment Officer. In those days, benefit fraud was rife, and was costing the country millions of pounds. Our job was to sort the wheat from the chaff, identify those in real need and weasel out the cheats. There was an astonishingly large number of malingerers, freeloaders, whingers and downright liars. We had several tricks up our sleeves to catch out the unwary.

'Did you manage to get parking all right? It's murder trying to find a space round here.'

'Oh, yes, doctor, I parked in the supermarket car park.'

That car park is 400 yards from the assessment centre. Claimants looking for mobility benefit should not be able to walk more than 200 yards.

Some claimants apparently suffered agonising and incapacitating back pain. They could hardly move. One of the tests which they had to endure was 'straight leg raising'. The claimant lies on their back on the couch, and the doctor attempts to raise a straight leg to 90 degrees, the theory being that true sufferers of sciatica will experience pain as the leg is raised and there is tension on the damaged nerve. Professional claimants have been fully briefed on this test and will start to yell and scream as soon as the leg is raised one centimetre. However, when asked to sit forwards so that the doctor can listen to the back of the chest, they do so with comparative ease. Sharp observers of geometry will have realised that this posture exactly replicates the 90 degree angle that proved impossible just a few minutes ago. Gotcha.

Amazing that people who simply cannot move the head in either direction, and who inevitably arrive wearing one of those ridiculous neck braces, will fall for the simple trap of 'what's this scar on your left shoulder?' Gotcha again.

There were numerous other ingenious traps for the unwary, but I will not describe them here, as you, dear reader, might just be one of those malingering whingers. Although I doubt it, as things have tightened up considerably in the benefits world.

The other sign of the coin features the truly disabled and incapacitated, deserving cases with appalling tales to tell of courage and fortitude in the face of genuine illness. One particular group that always touched my heart were the so-called FEPOWS – Far East Prisoners Of War. This dwindling group of former servicemen would be claiming pensions for injuries and illnesses sustained during their internment at the hands of the Japanese in World War 2. Many had worked on the railways, or in the jungles, most had suffered near starvation, beatings, torture, and on top of this contracted malaria, dengue fever, and other tropical diseases. They would often come to see me with drawings or handwritten accounts of their time in captivity. One poor man had a restraining order placed on him by the courts, preventing him from visiting mainline railway stations in London, as he had exhibited threatening behaviour towards Japanese tourists. He was so traumatised that he simply could not help himself and would break down in tears if there was any Japanese footage in a television programme, for example. All of these individuals were supposed to fill in all the claim forms for each disease or condition, but this never happened in practice. The word from the top was 'just give them everything', so they all ended up with a richly deserved full pension.

Part 3

Drug company 'research'.

From time to time, we would be approached by pharmaceutical companies who were keen to involve us in a 'research' project. Why the inverted commas? Because mostly, these projects were thinly disguised marketing strategies. Consider the set-up. The company in question has, for example, a new asthma inhaler on the market. They want you to test it against the currently available brand leader. They will supply all the medication for the 'trial', you just have to recruit a few willing patients who are prepared to take part. Over a period of time, they dutifully take the medication and record their results, whether it be actual readings on their home peak flow meter (a device to measure the strength of your blowing – this will be low if you are tight-chested and wheezing) or something like the number of times they felt wheezy per day / week. You, in turn, would receive a fee – usually generous - for the work involved. At the end of the 'trial', the results are collated, and the company will (hopefully) publish the results. Now bear in mind that patients in trial settings behave differently from normal patients – because they are being 'monitored', because they have to fill in a booklet, and because they want to keep the doctor happy, they take the medication as prescribed. What's weird about that? Well, research shows that patients probably, at best, take about half the doses they are supposed to take – they forget, they can't be bothered, they can't find the inhaler, they feel OK on that day etc. Unsurprisingly, their results on the 'new' inhaler are much better, their readings are higher, they have less bouts of wheeziness, it must be a wonder drug! The trial is over, the drug company has disappeared into the mist, you have pocketed a wad of cash, but the patient now wants to change to the new (more expensive) inhaler. And who can blame them. So they win, you win, the company wins, and the bill is footed by the NHS. Good strategy. Now don't get me wrong, there is a huge amount of excellent, academic, properly scrutinised research undertaken in general practice. There is a general practice research network, and thanks to computerisation, a world leading database, that leads to serious publications in serious journals. This is far removed from the 'research' I am describing. Since my day, things have changed dramatically, and there has been a clamp-down on such shoddy marketing practices.

One project we did undertake was for a new migraine treatment. Migraine is a miserable complaint, with millions of sufferers in the UK. In the 1980s, treatments were fairly unsatisfactory, so anything that promised a real change was welcomed with open arms. We quickly realised that, instead of waiting for migraine sufferers to randomly turn up, so that they could be offered the chance to take part in the trial, it might be better to compile a list of patients with a migraine diagnosis, and write to them, offering a life-changing opportunity. It was a long list. We were inundated with replies. We set up special clinics on Saturday mornings to satisfy the demand. Fortunately, the treatment really did represent a shift in migraine care. The patients were delighted, the company was delighted, we were minted. Our drugs bill gave the chaps in medicine management a bit of a headache, though.

Part 4

A pain in the neck.

One day in 1997, James returned from a holiday in a highly agitated state. Whilst away, he had met a GP who was involved in medical assessment of whiplash cases. He was becoming very wealthy very quickly. We needed to look into it. The premise was simple. People were involved in a road traffic incident, they sustained injuries such as whiplash (pain in the neck caused by being thrown forwards and backwards when hit from behind), or back pain, or bruising. The insurance companies needed a doctor to examine the claimant, write a report, and the claim could be settled. Up until this point in time, these reports were largely compiled by consultant orthopaedic surgeons, who charged huge fees and produced unnecessarily elaborate reports. The insurance industry thought it was time for a change. Why not use (cheap) GPs to see the less serious cases, write a short and sensible report, everyone is happy. Less cost to the insurance companies, possibly cheaper insurance premiums, less bureaucracy, hurrah! Everyone is happy apart from the consultant orthopaedic surgeons, who have to settle for a smaller yacht. Who gives a stuff about them, pompous upstarts?

It transpired that there was more than enough work out there. Accident management companies were springing up everywhere, acting on behalf of the insurance companies, and keen to recruit GPs who were prepared to take on the work. We looked at the fees they were offering, and decided we we were prepared to take on the work. This shift also coincided with the new complaints culture, which encouraged everyone to make claims, no matter how trivial the injury. Within a couple of months, we were registered with a dozen accident management companies, the work was flooding in. We needed a secretary to organise the appointments, we needed rooms in which to see the clients, we needed a company name, we needed headed notepaper. As we each had a day off per week, we could handle a lot of work. Most GPs who were embarking on this path were seeing one or two cases a week, usually in their own surgeries, usually after work. Allotting half an hour per case, we were able to see about 14 clients per day. It was amazingly easy. Ninety per cent of the cases had whiplash injuries, the stories were always the same, the treatments were always the same. Our reports were always the same. The format was so repetitive, we could dictate whole reports by changing just a few details.

We had overlooked just one thing. Many of the payments were made to us when the case was settled, which might be some time after the appointment with the client. So, initial costs were high, in that we had to pay for room hire, travel, secretarial costs, postage, and so on, but we were invoicing large amounts in return. The problem was the lag phase between report and payment, because, as we later found out, the lovely people at HMRC tax you on invoices, not monies received. So during the first year, we had huge outgoings, no income, huge tax bill. We survived, but it was touch and go as to whether the house would have to be remortgaged.

Business was booming, we opened up other offices in remote locations, and travelling time increased. One day, a quietly spoken man turned up at the office, and said 'I want to show you something that might change your life.' He opened his laptop to show me the prototype of his report writing software. This magic tool wrote the reports for you, using drop down menus, and even produced the invoices. The reports and invoices could be sent directly to the companies, who were happy to accept electronic reports. We were to be the guinea pigs. Sceptical at first, we made several suggestions for changes to the software. Eventually, after several re-writes, the prototype became reality. The quietly spoken man launched the product, charging users a set fee per report. It became the industry standard within a couple of years, and he became a very wealthy, though still quietly spoken man.

All good things come to an end. The market became overcrowded, accident management companies were able to offer lower fees, the whole whiplash market got out of hand, with staged accidents, and fraudulent claims. Costs were rising, income was falling, it was time to think about calling a halt to all this. One day, a barrister for the opposition phoned me about my report.

'You prepared the report on Mr. Singh, who alleges he suffered a whiplash injury in an accident on August 12th?'

'Indeed I did.'

'Would you be prepared to change your report to say that no such injury ever occurred?'

'I don't see why I should. I saw the client, took his history, examined him, and submitted my report.'

'Would you be prepared to withdraw your report if it transpired that on August 12th, Mr Singh was in Mumbai, and not Manchester?'

'Ah.'

Never mind, we had ten good years before it all turned sour. After all, it was just a bit on the side.

The Grim Reaper

The Grim Reaper walks at a preferred speed of 0.82 metres per second. If you walk slower than that, he's gonna get you. This is not fanciful nonsense, it is based on actual research done in Australia, and published in the esteemed British Medical Journal. The researchers looked at 1700 elderly subjects living in Melbourne and compared their walking speed to their risk of dying. Those with walking speeds of less than 0.82 metre per second had a higher risk of dying. On the other hand, those with a walking speed of greater than 1.36 metres per second were unlikely to get caught. Moral of the tale –walk faster!

Being in a south coast seaside town with a large retired population, the Grim Reaper made frequent visits to our patients. He had a season ticket, you might say. Most of his visits were to be expected, very elderly frail people with multiple medical problems, they might as well have booked an appointment.

Some visits were unexpected, and to put it mildly, rather inconvenient. One of these occurred in the surgery itself. As I have described, the surgery is in a Victorian building on the seafront. The main entrance is through the front door, leading into the reception and waiting room, which is always crowded. The rear entrance leads to some steep steps opening onto a car park. On the day in question, a patient had arrived complaining of breathlessness on exertion. He was seen by one of my partners, who examined him, and decided he needed an ECG. She left the patient in the consulting room, to see if the nurse was free to do the test in the downstairs treatment room. On returning to the patient, it was clear that the Reaper had popped in. Attempts to resuscitate the patient proved futile. We were then faced with a dead body, occupying a consulting room, in the middle of a busy surgery, patients' appointments now delayed, no free rooms. We called the undertakers, who would come to the car park. We then had to station a receptionist outside each surgery door, holding on to the handle so that the patients could not leave, whilst two able-bodied GPs carried the corpse, with as much dignity as we could muster, into the coffee room to await collection. Fortunately it all went smoothly, apart from some queries from patients who found a receptionist hanging on to the door handle as they attempted to escape.

Another incident occurred when I was called out by the police to an apparent murder. The 'victim' lay on his bed, in a dimly-lit room. There was blood all over the bed, the carpet, the bedside table. A lot of blood. In all other respects, it might have looked like a scene from a Stephen King movie. But where was the motive. What about the murder weapon? The clue was the overwhelming smell of stale tobacco, and the overflowing ashtray on the bedside table. A quick look at the notes confirmed that this chap had been diagnosed with lung cancer a couple of months ago. I assumed (and was subsequently proved right at the autopsy) that his cancer had eroded into his carotid artery, and he had bled to death.

One of our GPs did a stint at the local hospice once a week, reviewing the patients, adjusting medications, checking blood results. There was, understandably, a smooth and efficient process to deal with the frequent deaths that occurred. The deceased would be discreetly transferred to the 'chapel', a private room in a quiet part of the hospice. The chapel had back doors opening to a secret parking space into which the undertakers hearse would arrive. The back doors would be opened, the body of the deceased transferred and taken away.

On this occasion, a perplexed and rather worried looking undertaker appeared on the ward.

'Erm, there's no body in the chapel.'

'Of course there is, we wheeled her in there twenty minutes ago.'

'No, there's just an empty bed.'

At this point, an element of panic sets in. What has happened to Mrs. Smith? Surely she really had passed away? She can't be wandering round the corridors? Everyone rushed into the chapel to inspect the empty bed. Then the answer presented itself. Mrs. Smith, in her final days, had been nursed on a pressure mattress, a sort of airbed which relieves the body from pressure points. In order to move the bed to the chapel, the air supply had been disconnected, the mattress had deflated, leaving the deceased under a stretched white sheet which gave the appearance of an empty bed. Phew.

Oooh doctor!

'Doctor, I want you

Ooh, my doctor wanna do

I can't get over you

Doctor, do anything that ya wanna do.'

So sings the inimitable Caro Emerald on her stunning album *Deleted scenes from the cutting room floor.*

The inference is that the female patient is smitten by the gorgeous male doctor and he can 'do anything he wants to do.'

Well, he can't. The General Medical Council takes a very dim view of such behaviour and Dr. Gorgeous is likely to find himself struck off the medical register if his behaviour is anything other than unerringly professional.

Rewind to the days of 'Carry on' films. The hapless Dr. Kilmore, played by Jim Dale, is gazing wide-eyed at the undeniably fine body of Barbara Windsor. Great hilarity all round. Ooh, er matron and all that. The reality is slightly less amusing. The doctor-patient relationship is built on trust and professionalism. The patient, who may be required to expose certain bodily parts to the doctor, has to have the utmost confidence that he or she is only interested in fact finding and examination, in order to arrive at a diagnosis. We know, sadly, from numerous cases in the press and in the media (even Hollywood – remember *The Hand that Rocks the Cradle*?) that this is not always the case. The rules are quite clear, and as one wit efficiently summarised them, 'you can make your mistress your patient, but you can't make your patient your mistress.' Not exactly the spirit of the rules, but near enough. But what of Dr. Gorgeous? Is he/ she not also at risk of finding themselves in a compromising position? Patients falling for their doctors is commonplace, so much so that there is a medical syndrome associated with the phenomenon – De Cleramboult's syndrome. It is quite understandable, the patient having had close and intimate conversations with a kind, empathetic individual who is trying to help. There might be regular contact within the privacy of the consulting room, and of course, the removal of clothing. I know of at least one GP whose life was made miserable by a stalker, to the extent that legal proceedings were needed to restrain the offender.

For myself, an episode early in my professional life shocked me to the core. It was whilst I was working on the medical wards during my GP training. One of the patients, a shy, withdrawn lady in her forties was being seen by me on a Friday afternoon.

'Janet, you seem very anxious today, is anything wrong?'

'Well, yes, it's just that....it's just....I don't know how to say it.'

'Take your time. What is it?'

'I don't know how to tell you..... I am being discharged tomorrow, and I wanted you to come and spend the weekend with me.'

I was absolutely speechless. My mouth opened, but no words came out. Eventually, I muttered something and escaped from the ward. When I explained to the nursing staff what had happened, there were knowing smiles, the occasional giggle.

'Didn't you know she fancies you? Isn't it obvious? She only puts on make-up when you are around.'

I was completely unaware of this information, and shocked, and indeed angry, that the staff knew all about this, and had not bothered to inform me, when a vulnerable patient was involved. I had to inform the consultant. He was very sanguine about the whole thing.

'Yes, yes, typical case of transference. I'll just make sure she doesn't see you again.'

And that was that. Janet was discharged from the hospital, and I have no idea what became of her.

Another patient, a divorced lady in her fifties, was a frequent visitor to the surgery, with depression. On more than one occasion, she said 'I think I would feel better if I was getting some sex.' She would then glance, not at all shyly, in my direction. I think she thought that the answer to her medical problems would be available on the NHS. It was not to be.

It was common practice, and indeed the recommendation of the General Medical Council, and the medical defence organisations, to offer a chaperone for any procedures that might compromise a patient, or indeed the doctor. There were also large notices in every consulting room, clearly stating that it was the right of the patient, male or female, to request the presence of a chaperone at any time. Despite this, I can recall less than a dozen occasions when the offer was taken up.

'Don't be silly, doctor, you've known me for years.'

'You've seen it all before, doc.'

This was indeed true, and it was a measure of the trust that existed, that there was no awkwardness in the everyday performance of my medical duties, no matter what orifice was being examined. Many health care professionals, and many patients, have also stated that the presence of a chaperone actually increases the embarrassment, as there is an implicit suggestion that neither is to be trusted. In any event, the increase in cases of litigation has reached such a level that you would be mad not to offer, even insist upon, a chaperone, and document in the medical record any refusal.

What's in a name?

There is a website which lists some of the most difficult to pronounce words in the English language. They include *anathema*, *isthmus* and *phenomenon*. Curiously missing, however, is the one which seems to crop up daily in general practice - Ibuprofen. This commonly used anti-inflammatory drug has, over the years, accumulated a dozen or so aliases;

-ibubrufen (paying homage to its original trade name (Brufen)

-iburofen

-ifubropen

-ibufen

-ipobroben

I do not possess a decent singing voice, but when asked for 'some Galveston', I am tempted to rattle off a few verses of the Glen Campbell classic, rather than to dispense a bottle of that pink gloopy heartburn remedy.

'I feel a bit nethalgic, doctor.' I know exactly what they mean, but this unwitting fusion of the words 'lethargic' and 'nostalgic' is used so commonly that it is in danger of creeping into the Oxford English Dictionary. I suppose the definition would be something like 'to have a fond remembrance of what it once felt like to be weary.'

'My heart was beating ten to the dozen.' (What? Slower than normal?)

In my early years in the practice, I looked after a charming elderly lady called Decima. I once enquired as to the origins of her name. 'Look at my date of birth' she said. She was born on the 10th October 1910. 10 10 10. Her father was a maths teacher, she explained.

People should really take some time to consider the implications of the name they give their child.

I am conducting a post-natal visit, to check that everything is OK, and to complete the paperwork to register the child with the practice.

'And what name have you chosen for your new son?'

'Tyson' the parents reply in unison.

If this boy should turn out to be a weedy bespectacled genius, who goes on to found a social media empire, then Tyson might be a tad inappropriate. If however, this same boy should turn out to be a slow-witted, obese, violent thug who will become familiar with the layout of a prison cell, then Tyson might be indeed applicable.

I take a long hard look at both parents.

'Good choice' I say.

A touch of the vapours

I feel that I must start this section with a huge disclaimer.

I am in no way suggesting that the conditions described in this part of the book are fake, made up, imagined or illusory. Furthermore, I am not suggesting that *most* people who suffer from these conditions do not have real symptoms and real suffering, bringing misery to their lives.

Is that clear? Good.

However, you may be aware that of all the people who give their faith, in surveys or censuses, as *Church of England*, less than half actually go to church. What I am suggesting is that things are not always what they seem, and that not all those who give their condition as, for example, ME, are worshippers at that particular altar, if you see what I mean.

In Victorian times, ladies would often swoon for fairly trivial reasons, possibly following a remark of a sexual nature, and they were said to have 'the vapours' - a reference to the smelling salts used to revive them, usually provided by a dashing young gentleman.

Neurasthenia was a concept introduced in 1869, by neurologist George Millar Beard. Sufferers had lassitude, fatigue, and irritability occurring in the absence of objective cause. Sigmund Freud blamed it on sexual excess, but then he would, wouldn't he? It is no longer regarded as a diagnosis by the American Psychiatry Association.

Next up is myalgic encephalomyelitis, or ME, which tends to get lumped together with CFS, chronic fatigue syndrome, or PVFS, post-viral fatigue syndrome. All of these conditions are characterised by easy fatiguability, muscle weakness, mental exhaustion, insomnia, headaches, cognitive dysfunction, and so on.

More recently, there were moves to link these conditions to Candida. Candida is a yeast which lives naturally in the human intestine, but 'overgrowth' has been blamed for many things, including ME, the usual culprit for the shift in balance being overuse of antibiotics in modern medicine.

(*Candida* was also a hit song in the 1970s by Dawn, who you will remember also recorded *Tie a yellow ribbon round the old oak tree.* I don't think *Candida* would make it into the charts today, even if sung by the charming Ed Sheeran.)

The common thread linking all these conditions is that the symptoms are vague, physical signs are few, if any, and there are no diagnostic tests. Treatments are often unsatisfactory or unhelpful. Now if you are a sufferer from any of the above conditions, that seems very depressing. You can't have a ME blood test, or a scan to confirm that this is the cause of your troubling symptoms. Traditional medicine cannot seem to offer you any hope, or specific treatments. But don't worry, there are plenty of 'alternative' treatments to solve your problem, usually without a shred of evidence to support their outrageous claims.

Now, you might be inclined to think that the above information could lead to allegations of fabrication and malingering. Sadly, this is so. ME has been called 'the malingerer's disease', scorn has been poured on the stories of many sufferers, suggestions have been made that what they really need is a brisk walk round the block, or some good fresh air, or a proper job.

My experience is mixed. I have known many genuine cases, I have also known other cases where the diagnosis was 'convenient', allowing the individual to avoid work, or school, or to claim benefits. One young man I recall, the son of a midwifery colleague, developed ME shortly after starting university. The condition dragged on for a couple of years, his parents consulted all manner of quacks, spent fortunes on hopeless remedies. Whenever I saw him in the surgery, I would look him in the eye, and I would see deception, and a certain smugness. He made a dramatic recovery when his benefits were stopped by a wise assessment officer.

Another case was that of a super-fit athlete, a runner and cyclist, who developed ME after glandular fever (a well-known trigger) and who took over a year to recover. I have seldom seen such desperation and frustration as he fought against this most stubborn foe.

Something I am reluctant to throw in to the mix is PTSD – post-traumatic stress disorder. This term came to prominence in relation to American soldiers returning from the conflict in Vietnam. In earlier days it might have been called 'shell shock'. The term has now grown to encompass other traumatic life events such as sexual assault, mugging, road traffic accidents, any event which is life-threatening. It is characterised by severe anxiety, flashbacks, insomnia, extreme irritability or jumpiness. The trouble is that this term has been hijacked by certain individuals who clearly do not suffer from PTSD, and to some extent, this is disrespectful to real sufferers, especially perhaps those in the armed forces.

So, to clarify; if you have been serving in Afghanistan and the vehicle ahead of you in the convoy is blown up by a roadside bomb, you are entitled to suffer from PTSD. Similarly, if you have been staring down the barrel of a gun, as some thug relieves you of your wallet, you would have a valid claim. You do not have PTSD if someone bumps into your car in Tesco car park. You do not have PTSD if someone says you look a bit overweight on Facebook. There was a famous spat when Piers Morgan accused a well-known pop star of suffering from WNTS – weedy nerdy twerp syndrome, rather than the PTSD he claimed he had been suffering from. I have some sympathy with his views on the subject, despite the fact that I can't stand the man. Similarly, in my practice, I have dealt with several cases of PTSD and er, WNTS.

Levels of evidence

As doctors we are encouraged to practice evidence- based medicine. That is, we are directed to ensure that any intervention, be it a medicine, a surgical procedure, a course of therapy, has the best possible evidence base to support its application. There are different levels of evidence, from strongest to weakest. This is termed the hierarchy of evidence. At the top is the randomised controlled trial, then systematic review of available evidence, then case studies, and finally expert opinion. So, in the absence of good data from trials and studies, the *weakest* form of evidence that is acceptable is the opinion of the leading experts in the field. Think about that. To come back for an instant to the randomised controlled trial. This is a study in which a number of similar people are randomly assigned to 2 (or more) groups to test a specific drug, treatment or other intervention. One group (the experimental group) has the intervention being tested, the other (the comparison or control group) has an alternative intervention, a dummy intervention (placebo) or no intervention at all. The groups are followed up to see how effective the experimental intervention was. Outcomes are measured at specific times and any difference in response between the groups is assessed statistically. At the end of the trial, there is only considered to be statistically significant between the treatments if there is less than a 1 in 20 chance that the results did not occur by chance. A very good result occurs when there is less than a 1 in 100 probability that the results occurred by chance. All very interesting, I hear you say, between yawns, but why are you telling us this?

The next time you see a shampoo advertisement on the telly, have a close look at the screen. 'Shinyshine shampoo gives you the shiniest hair!!' screams the banner headline, as the gorgeous model tosses her head, sending her gorgeous silky, bouncy hair swirling across the screen. (Does anyone ever actually do that in the real world?). But in tiny letters at the bottom of the screen, it says '70% of 93 women agreed'. Hold it there. These women will, in all probability, have been given the shampoo to try free of charge, the bottles will be labelled Shinyshine shampoo. The participants will want to please the sponsor. They might have had a day out in London. And in spite of all this, 30% did NOT agree that their hair was the shiniest ever. And are you telling me that mega-companies like L'Oreal or Proctor and Gamble, who manufacture these products, can only afford to survey 93 people?? Not good enough.

And of course, patients have their own hierarchy of evidence. At the top is *my mate Sharon*.

'You know those pills you put me on, doctor, well, my mate Sharon says they don't work. Her friend was on them and she said they were rubbish.'

Next level – the woman in the post office. Personally, I think she has the intellectual edge over the woman in the wool shop. I don't know what it is, perhaps she has studied more texts, had a broader range of experience, but my money is on her. And she sometimes gets it right. 'That doesn't sound right to me, love, it could be your thyroid, I'd see the doctor if I were you.' Correct. Shame they can't hand out thyroid pills with the stamps and benefits. The way things are going with the NHS, that might be a viable option.

Even my own dear mother is not immune.

'I've got crusty skin on my ear. My hairdresser says it's cancer.'

Her hairdresser, for God's sake, I bet she hasn't even ever worked in a post office.

'Your hairdresser says it's cancer, does she? Which medical school did she go to?'

'Don't be like that.'

'Mum, I've seen your crusty skin and it's not cancer.'

'Are you sure?'

I am sure, because she has *chondrodermatitis helicis chronica*, an irritating condition with an implausibly long name, but not cancerous. Yet my mother would doubt the word of her own son, a fully qualified doctor, in favour of someone who spends their day twiddling curlers and dispensing blue rinses.

Next level – *The Daily Mail*. At this point, I pour myself a nice glass of red wine, even though yesterday's headline told me I was definitely going to die, if I finish it. *The Daily Mail* is, I am informed, the second most widely read daily after *the Sun*. Some people with a long memory will recall that during the war, it was pro-Hitler and pro-fascist, a historical fact it has struggled to shrug off or conceal. But move on, let's forgive and forget, we all make mistakes, after all. But the *Daily Mail* makes more mistakes than most. Even in recent times, it has been accused of racism, sexism, homophobia, and of failing to maintain basic standards of accuracy and accountability. Even Wikipedia has condemned *The Mail* as an 'unreliable source' to use as a reference on its site. It has been accused of printing sensationalist and inaccurate scare stories of science and medical research.

It is also decidedly anti-doctor. Pick up a copy (and I mean pick up, from a waste bin or a park bench, don't spend good money on it), and I can guarantee you that you won't make it to page 12 without some story like 'Doctors failed to diagnose my cancer until it was too late' or 'grabbing GPs to get extra slice of NHS cash for doing nothing'. Check it out.

So, despite this, a lot of patients still believe what they are reading. They used to arrive at appointments clutching neatly trimmed clippings from the paper, about cancer scares, miracle cures, mystical healers, secret research. If you have the time, Google *Daily Mail* and Cancer. There is a website called www.anorak.co.uk that lists alphabetically all the things that *the Mail* has linked with cancer. It includes baby food, candle-lit dinners, left-handedness, and Worcester sauce.

My particular beef with this paper is the stories it ran on statins (cholesterol lowering drugs). The misinformation and inaccuracies may have led many readers to stop taking their tablets, thereby increasing the risk of heart attack and stroke.

I recall a question I was asked at a medical conference;

'I have been prescribed simvastatin, but the Daily Mail says it will cause cancer.'

'Then you should definitely stop taking it.'

'Simvastatin?'

'No, The Daily Mail.'

And finally, the (fairly) new kid on the block, Google.

I really don't have a problem with Google, although I used to shudder when the newspaper clippings were superseded by reams of printouts from bizarre websites. A lot of the information is useful, but there are dangers. For example, if you have a little too much wine, then nod off in front of the telly, you might wake some hours later, with a stiff neck and a headache. Google this, and you will find, to your horror, that you not only have a grim hangover, but you have developed meningitis to go with it. American websites are best avoided, as they tend to be commercialised, and written by faux medics called Hyram Strifemberg the third.

Tales from the surgery

I am called out one evening to a rather rowdy pub on the seafront. A darts match is in progress. Unfortunately, one of the participants, who has the usual athletic appearance of a dart player, has collapsed, and is lying on the darts mat surrounded by anxious faces. The patient is grey and sweaty, and I diagnose a heart attack. An ambulance is called. I check his pulse and blood pressure, resisting the overwhelming temptation to shout out 'One hundred and eighty'. As we await the arrival of the ambulance, one of the dart players leans in and asks 'Do you think it would be safe to move him?' For an instant, I am touched by his concern for the comfort of his fellow athlete, until he adds 'only we've got a game on'.

Geraldine is a 50 year old lady who presented with palpitations, and was subsequently diagnosed as suffering from a heart valve problem, so serious it warranted surgery to replace the damaged valve. This solves the immediate problem, but she is left with an irregular heartbeat. To cheer herself up after the surgery, she has arranged an evening at the local concert hall. The man sitting immediately behind her in the audience is clearly agitated. Eventually, he taps her on the shoulder and asks 'Is it you making that infernal clicking noise?' 'Yes', she replies proudly, 'it's my new metal heart valve.' 'Well, could you at least try to make it beat in time to the music?' he demands.

Anne is a former nurse who initially presented with a bowel disturbance. She was referred to the specialist, who organised a barium enema. For those of you unaware of this procedure it involves pumping a large volume of a chalky liquid into the lower bowel. Being radio-opaque, it allows x-rays to be taken which can demonstrate defects in the wall of the bowel. Unfortunately, it can take some time to expel the thick, white material after the procedure. Anne came to see me 3 days later, complaining of constipation. I urged patience. I saw her again a few days later and enquired about her progress. She told me that shortly after seeing me, she was to attend a dinner party hosted by some rather posh friends. The house was modern and open-plan. Half way through the meal, she realised to her horror that the barium was about to make its long overdue reappearance. She excused herself and went to the toilet, which was just off the dining area. After her performance, she glanced down, and was alarmed to see, as she herself put it, about a dozen white billiard balls bouncing on the surface. She flushed. They bounced back. After a respectable time, she flushed again. They bounced back. It was time to take her place once more at the table. 'What on earth did you do?' I enquired. 'I did what any sensible person would do' she replied, 'I fished them all out, wrapped them in toilet paper, and took them home in my handbag.'

I am confronted by a nervous man, who is taking rather a long time to get to the point. Eventually he stutters 'Well, doctor, the problem is this. My wife and I are unable to have refreshments.' I am wondering why his culinary problems are my concern, when I realise he is actually describing sexual impotence.

A holidaymaker pitches up at the surgery in an emergency appointment.

'How can I help you?'

'Well doctor, I injured my wrist yesterday, and I'm going home today. How am I going to carry my suitcase?'

'Carry it with the other hand.'

'Ok, doc, thank you.'

Five years at medical school were not wasted after all.

Lena, one of our senior nurses, is seeing a patient in the treatment room for a routine blood pressure check. Ever vigilant, she notices something unusual in the medical record.

'I can't find any record of your having a cervical smear test,'

'You won't. I've never had one.'

'But that's terrible. You should be having them regularly. Look, I'm not busy at the moment, why don't we just pop you up on the couch and do it now?'

'I don't think I need one,'

'Don't be silly, it'll only take a minute.'

'No, I mean I have been told I will never need one.'

'Why's that?'

'Because I have had a gender reassignment.'

'What do you mean?'

(remember, this was in the days when LGBT stood for Loves Getting Book Tokens)

'Well, I used to be a man, but they removed my penis, then turned my scrotum inside out to make a false vagina.'

Never has the literary phrase 'she ran screaming from the room' seemed applicable to a general practice situation.

I am confronted by a young man wearing ludicrously striped trousers and an offensive T-shirt. He swaggered into the consulting room, and declared, without preamble, 'My girlfriend says my sperm tastes funny'. I was temporarily discombobulated, but quickly regained my composure. 'I am assuming she is a connoisseur?' I retorted. This took the wind out of his sails, so I followed up with 'it might be an infection in your prostate gland. We need to send off a sample of your sperm. Perhaps your girlfriend could bring the sample up to the lab?' ' In this pot' I then added, lest there be any confusion.

A slovenly girl, concentrating on her chewing gum, slumps in the chair.

'I think I've got thrust.'

'I think you mean thrush' I opine, whilst thinking 'but I'm sure thrust was a causative factor.'

Hypochondriacs are a common feature of general practice. There are those with a genuine phobia of illness, those who think every itch and twitch is a sign of impending death, those who make the most of minor illnesses, or who always seem to be in the throes of 'something that's going round'. And there are people like Mike.

Mike is a friend as well as patient - a retired successful businessman, a reformed alcoholic. He never shies away from telling you about his drinking days, when he would consume several bottles of white wine per day. He is overweight, smokes too much, and is subject to stress. He is loud, bombastic, and always speaks his mind. He was a frequent surgery attender. A harmless mole on his back. 'It's cancer, isn't it, just tell me how long I've got, be straight with me.' A twinge in the loin. 'It's my kidneys, isn't it? What are my chances of a transplant?'

One day, he rang me at home. I was out, so he spoke to my wife, who was well used to his habits.

'Tell him I've got bowel cancer.'

'Righto, Mike, will do.'

The phone rang again thirty minutes later.

'Mike here. Tell him not to worry, I haven't got bowel cancer.'

'That was a quick cure.'

'Well it was like this. This morning, I passed a whole lot of blood in the toilet. That's when I rang Eugene, but he wasn't in, so I spoke to my sister, who used to be a nurse. She asked me if I had eaten anything unusual. Then I remembered that, the previous day, I had bought a pack of six cooked beetroot. The first one was so delicious, that I had another, and before I knew it, I had finished off the lot. So, it's OK after all.'

Mike would then recount this tale at dinner parties, to the amusement of the whole table. Rather disconcertingly, he was also fond of pointing at me and saying 'there's only two people in the world who've had their finger in my bum, and he's one of them.' No-one dared ask about the other one.

One of my diabetic patients asks whether it is true that cinnamon can lower blood sugar. This is actually true, but the amount that needs to be ingested is quite large – about two teaspoons per day. I am impressed that she has done the research, but my admiration is immediately offset by her cinnamon-containing list, which includes apple pies and donuts. I have always wanted to use the Jimmy Carr line about people who attribute their weight gain to 'thyroid problems'. His reply is 'what are you treating it with – pies?' Never dared.

I am attempting to listen to the sorry litany of woes that make up the life of Sharon, but it is difficult, as her two brats are making a fairly good job of dismantling my surgery. They jump on the examination couch, they open drawers and cupboards. It is only when they start taking syringes and needles from one of the drawers that she turns a weary face towards them and says 'Wayne. Don't.' It is said without conviction, and fails to elicit any response from Wayne, so I am forced to intervene, firmly closing the drawers and glaring menacingly at them.

'Do you ever smack your children?' I ask.

'Oh, no, never, doctor.'

'Well, perhaps you should.'

An hour later, I am being lectured to by an irate health visitor.

KGB – a motley assortment of nameless, faceless individuals, and who spy on you constantly, then report back to their superiors in a tyrannical regime. Feared by all, they scrutinise, criticise, and mete out terrible punishments.

CQC – see above.

Just joking. Well almost.

The CQC – Care Quality Commission monitors, inspects and regulates social care services. Their duties include inspection of general practice premises to ensure quality and safety.

At least they give you notice of their arrival, giving the practice adequate time to ensure that all these rigorous standards are met – there are up-to-date policy documents, all supplies and medications are in date, clinical governance has been adhered to, everything is spotless.

On the wall behind my desk, there is a shelf on which I kept a few nick-nacks. There was a collection of old cameras, a 1920s textbook of medicine, a couple of teddy bears, some juggling balls. This provided a distraction, a talking point, and was infinitely preferable to a boring collection of medical texts. I was quite fond of it, but it did encourage a little dust to settle in its hiding places. The CQC visit was imminent. The practice manager arrives one day with a large cardboard box and politely suggests that I clear my shelf, and replace the contents with boring medical texts. I start to protest, but realise it is futile, and set about my task.

'Oh, and another thing' she says. The CQC visit is scheduled for a day in which I will be in the surgery. The suggestion is made that I might like to swap days with someone who won't call them the KGB, be deliberately obtuse, make inappropriate jokes, and be generally obstructive. I can see the sense in this.

The day arrives, the inspection occurs, interviews take place, fingers run along dust-free shelves. We eventually learn that we have been rated as GOOD, and everyone is thrilled. Except me. Why have we not been rated as OUTSTANDING? Are we not an outstanding practice? We provide an excellent service, the patients all think we are wonderful, we reach all our targets. I am informed that we cannot be OUTSTANDING because;

a) We don't have a lift. We don't have a lift because we have been forced to practice from a 19th century seaside villa, with no hope of moving. Every time we got to the top of the list for new premises, the government changed, or the healthcare system, and we went back to the end of the queue.

b) We aren't a training practice. We aren't a training practice because we have been forced to practice from a 19th century seaside villa, with insufficient space for the doctors and nurses, let alone an aspiring GP.

GOOD will have to be good enough.

My next patient is a chubby girl in her 20s, who presents with a two-week history of intermittent lower abdominal pain.

'Pop up on the couch' I say, and she duly does.

My brief examination instantly locates the source of the troublesome pains. She is, by my estimation, about 36 weeks pregnant. I gently break the glad (?) tidings, and she is utterly shocked. She resolutely denies all knowledge of her condition, stating that she thought that her weight gain was down to too many chocolates and crisps.

This is not an isolated case. There are dozens of reports in the literature of women arriving at the surgery at various stages of pregnancy, *even in labour*, who deny any possibility that they could be about to produce some offspring. Having watched my own wife endure two pregnancies, coloured as they were with morning sickness, heartburn, kicks, cramps and early contractions, I find it impossible to believe that cases like the one above could occur. (I was going to say inconceivable, but thought better of it.)

Any did I use the word 'chubby' to describe the appearance of that young girl? Hush my mouth! We are not allowed to use such derogatory terms any more. I hark back to a website I came across some time ago, featuring real American magazine advertisements from the 50s and 60s. In addition to shops selling clothes for 'chubby children', there were intimations that you were not a real man unless you smoked Camel cigarettes, and the helpful suggestion that if I wanted to make my wife thrilled and happy on Christmas morning, I should buy her a Hoover. I have the suspicion that, were I to do so, I would feature in the section of this book called *Things in places they shouldn't oughta be.*

And now, confronted with any patient weighing over 20 stones (or the equivalent in kilograms) I am not allowed to use the word 'fat'. Even *obese*, the technically correct term attracts disapproving frowns. No, they are indeed *nutritionally challenged* or some such bollocks. Even fat people call themselves fat.

I'm a celebrity

Given the ever-increasing numbers of A-list, B-list and C-list celebrities, it would be somewhat unusual to go through a career in general practice without encountering at least one, in a professional capacity. There have been several once-famous sitcom actors, a couple of politicians (they all have to live somewhere), and assorted musicians.

One day, the practice received a phone call from a local hotel;

'Would a doctor be able to call in and see one of our residents today?'

'We would normally expect the patient to make their way to the surgery. We can fit them in at 11.00 this morning.'

'The resident can't come to the surgery, I'm afraid.'

'Is he elderly or infirm?'

'No.'

'Confined to bed?'

'No.'

'Contagious?'

'No.'

'Well, then he can come down to the surgery.'

'No, he can't.'

'Why not?'

'Because he's...he's Simon Sparkle.' (Not his real name, of course, but you get the drift.)

The conversation was relayed to me, and I agreed to visit. Not that I was starstruck, you understand, nor a fan of Simon Sparkle (more of a T.Rex follower myself), but I was undeniably intrigued.

I arrived at the hotel, and was directed to the Sparkle suite. A brick-built security man stood guard.'

'Oo are you?' he demanded.

I was wearing my best corduroy jacket with elbow patches, and carrying a doctor's bag, but obviously, further identification was required.

'I'm the doctor. I have come to visit Mr. Sparkle.' (I hardly know the man, first name terms seemed a little premature.)

Without breaking his stare, he rapped his hairy knuckles on the door behind him.

'Simon, it's the doctor.'

I was shown into a large bedroom where Mr. Sparkle, naked to the waist, was having his bouffant locks teased into his trademark coiffe. He immediately got to his feet and proffered a hand.

'Hi, I'm Simon Sparkle.'

'Yes, I know.'

I dealt speedily with his minor musculoskeletal complaint (hardly surprising you might sprain your ankle stomping about in great platform boots like that), and left with two tickets for his show (unwanted) and a signed photo (unasked for).

A doctor I trained with was working as a junior hospital doctor in London, and was looking after a female 1960s pop star, when he received a phone call enquiring about her progress. Naturally cautious about bogus calls from the paparazzi, he replied that he was unable to discuss such matters over the phone.

'If you are indeed a friend of hers, you can visit at an appropriate hour.'

'I can't, I'm afraid, I'm calling from New York.'

The voice sounded familiar.

'Who is this?'

'It's John Lennon.' And it was.

Later in my career, I was asked to do a stint on an 'expert diabetes panel' for a pharmaceutical company training video. It was to be filmed in the National motorcycle museum in Birmingham, and was to be chaired by none other than Dr. Hilary Jones. We all arrived the previous night, and had dinner in a nearby hotel, after which we discussed the running order for the following day. At breakfast, the producer said to me 'You've come up here by car, haven't you? Perhaps you could take Hilary to the venue?' I wasn't in a position to refuse, but was horrified at the prospect, as my beaten up old Renault badly needed a wash, and I knew it would be full of empty crisp packets and Coke tins courtesy of my teenage kids. To make matters worse, I had parked the car under a tree in the hotel car park, and overnight the entire avian population of Birmingham had used it as a toilet. So instead of a nice black shiny Mercedes limo, the famed doctor was to be transported in an aged, faded, litter-strewn, bird-shit festooned banger. Hilary took it all in his stride, and we joked about it as we set off. However, the motorway network in that part of the world is fiendishly complicated, and as Hilary was telling me about his new swimming pool, I became distracted, and missed a crucial junction. I tried to rectify my mistake, but the correct carriageway was now at a standstill. It was a warm day, no air-conditioning in my car, so we wound the windows down as we edged along in the jam. We could see the astonished glances of fellow motorists, as they struggled to convince themselves that 'that doctor from the telly' was indeed travelling in such style. I can only assume that they had to put it down to an amazing look-alike. We arrived at the venue with minutes to spare before our allotted slot. The producer was pacing up and down outside the building, fuming and swearing. We went into the studio, where, ten minutes later, Dr. Hilary Jones, appeared in front of the cameras.

'Welcome to the first of a series of talks from experts in the field of diabetes.'

Word-perfect, polished, unflustered, despite his traumatic experience. Star quality.

Significant others

General practitioners do not function in isolation. They depend heavily on a team which includes not only the staff of the practice, but attached staff, and others working in the community. In 1985, this was sort of an extended family. In 2015, it was more like a bunch of disparate individuals, all with targets, clinical governance, budgets, and petty politics to cope with.

<u>The practice staff</u>

This lovely group was headed by the practice manager. In those far off days, most practice managers were upgraded nurses, who did the books, took the minutes at practice meetings, and organised cleaners. Nowadays, the practice manager will have a background in business, with a degree or two, and be fully conversant with pensions, employment law, counter fraud measures, as well as the never-ending tomes of rules and targets put out almost weekly by the commissioning bodies. My first practice manager was a busy woman of short stature. She knew how to keep the doctors in check, sort out petty squabbles amongst the receptionists, organise the practice nursing staff, and keep a good supply of biscuits in the coffee room. When she retired, we thought it was time we moved on to the new style of manager. We recruited a formidable businesswoman, who expected instant decisions on the future of the practice, rather than the 'shall we move this on to the next practice meeting agenda?' sort of approach we sometimes adopted. One day she took me to task for undercharging a patient for a taxi medical.

'It's a lot of money, and I know he can't really afford it, so I charged him half' was my defence.

'Are you running a business here, or a charity?' was her retort.

By our very nature, we are a bunch of softies, with innate knowledge of our patients, and a large dose of compassion.

She didn't last long.

Practice nurses.

1985 – cuts and bruises, leg ulcers, taking out stitches.

2015 – most run specialist clinics for diabetes, asthma, contraception, heart disease, travel medicine, in fact most of what a 1985 GP would have spent his or her time doing. In addition, there are practice nurse consultants, who see patients, prescribe drugs, diagnose and refer.

Attached staff.

This used to include mainly district nurses and health visitors, but nowadays is more likely to also feature in-house pharmacists, counsellors, and 'care navigators' who help patients through the maze of modern health care, benefits, post-operative care, and so on. Our district nurses used to be 'our' nurses. They knew us and the patients well, and would 'pop in' to see us during surgery to say 'just been out to see Ethel, leg ulcer looks a bit infected, could you check on it when you're out?' or 'Fred was looking a bit peaky this morning, so I checked his blood pressure, it was a bit up, just thought I'd let you know.' Now, we have teams, and the district nurse might come from a different town. Their time is strictly monitored, so much per visit, and record keeping is a more urgent priority than having a chat and a cup of tea with a lonely patient (those cups of tea often yielded vital information about the patient or illness that would not otherwise have surfaced).

Pharmacists

These used to be the chaps called 'chemists' who translated your illegible hand-written prescription into a bottle of pills. Now, they are likely to be based in the practice, monitoring every acute and repeat prescription for safety, appropriateness, dangerous interactions, as well as possible abuse, and of course, cost. Vital.

Counsellors

I used to think that counsellors were airy-fairy types who spouted a load of mumbo-jumbo. How my views changed! I now see them as a vital part of general practice, helping people with anxiety, depression, bereavement issues and so much more.

Chiropractors and osteopaths

Yes, I do know that they are different.

Contrary to popular belief, I have nothing against this breed of professionals. I just wish they would change their chat-up lines. Without fail, every patient who took themselves off with back pain, or hip pain, or even a headache was told that they had a 'tilted pelvis' or 'one leg longer than the other.'

Also, I am not sure I would want my back or neck violently twisted by someone who had not had the benefit of looking at an X-ray to reassure themselves that there isn't a spinal fracture or a secondary cancer which is causing the pain.

Homeopaths

A largely harmless bunch of people, with no evidence whatsoever to back up their claims. They do, however, seems to make an inordinate amount of money from selling atoms.

Spiritualists, soothsayers, and crystal merchants

Anyone who tells you that they can establish a communication with your recently departed loved one is deluded and cruel.

Locums

Locums, as I am sure you know, are those lovely people who step in to fill a vacancy in the practice caused by illness, maternity leave, holidays, or more likely these days, failure to recruit a new partner. They come in various shapes and sizes, and varying levels of ability. Over the years, we have had some interesting characters. The one I remember most clearly is Graham. In the pre-computer age, pathology results from the hospital (blood tests, urine tests) came on little pieces of paper. These were then passed to the doctors to assess, and mark as 'normal', 'abnormal', 'repeat', 'urgent' or 'see patient'. The audit process allowed us to see which doctor had been sent which result to deal with. With a worrying frequency, Graham would tick abnormal results as 'normal'. This would eventually come to light and be dealt with more appropriately. We decided to confront Graham with some of these reports. His response? 'That's not my tick.'

Again, before computers were trained to do the task, one of the most onerous and boring general practice tasks was the completion of medical reports for insurance companies, the so-called PMAs (personal medical assessments. This was well-paid work, and was designed to inform the companies issuing life insurance whether their client. John Smith, was likely to live for forty days or forty years before they had to pay out. However, this often meant sorting through hundreds of pages of illegible script, tattered folded hospital letters, referral notes, and letters from patients, all in the wrong chronological order. In order to ensure fairness, these tasks were doled out equally and fairly by the practice manager. Any tardiness in completion would lead to a letter from the insurance company requesting a more immediate attitude. The letters dramatically increased in frequency after the arrival of Graham.

'Have you done that report for Lifelong Assurance, Graham? They are chasing it.'

'Oh, that one, I sent it back weeks ago.'

The situation worsened, with strong letters now bearing the hint of legal action. Eventually, a receptionist, looking for a piece of medical equipment, opened a cupboard in Graham's office, and Tom and Jerry style, was buried in hundreds of hidden insurance report folders which avalanched down on top of her. The game was up, and Graham moved on to pastures new, in Siberia, or Scunthorpe, I believe.

Greta was an Eastern European doctor, who joined us for a couple of years. She had many talents. She spoke several languages. She had come third in a paella cooking competition in Spain. But the thing that impressed us the most was her expertise in substance abuse. She readily took on the patients with drug and alcohol abuse, some of whom were, shall we say, mildly threatening figures. It was not at all unusual for a heavily pierced and tattooed individual to turn up in her surgery, asking for a variety of substances. Unphased, she would thrust a urine container at them.

'Go and fill this.'

She would then put the sample into a diabolically clever little machine, wait a few minutes, then announce;

'Your urine sample shows that in the last 48 hours you have consumed diazepam, cannabis, and methadone. You are not entitled to any of the medications you request. Now get out.'

Had it been me, I would have been terrified that they would make a violent lunge at me, or produce a weapon, or, at the very least, hurl obscene abuse at me. But Greta would fix them with a stare that confirmed that the consultation was at an end, and they would slink, tail between legs, down the corridor.

It wasn't me

Whilst I can attest that 95% of the accounts in this book are a true record of my experiences, and opinions, there remains a section that deserves inclusion, but for which I cannot, and perhaps would not wish to, claim responsibility. Some of what follows did occur in my own practice, some has been reported to me by colleagues from elsewhere. But the one common thread is that fact that *it wasn't me.*

Agnes Poole was a serial home visit requester. We were all familiar with her irritating Scottish accent (other Scottish accents are available), her pleading dialogue, her wizened pain-contorted features. She truly believed that it was her divine right to have a GP visit her at home, rather than make it to an appointment at the surgery. Most of her calls were for trivial complaints, or even for a repeat prescription. Our reception staff had long ago given up all hope of convincing her to come down, and simply passed the calls on to us.

One day, the visiting doctor was at the end of his tether.

'Mrs. Poole, you do realise that this visit was entirely unnecessary. You could have come to the surgery. You have wasted my time, time that could have been better spent visiting someone who truly needed to be seen at home.'

'Oh, I don't know how you can say that, doctor, after all, I'm a cancer patient.' More facial contortions, more pathetic hand-wringing, the irritating voice now reduced to a pitiful whisper.

'You are no more a cancer patient than I am, Mrs. Poole. You had cancer twenty years ago, it was dealt with, you are cured, and you no longer have any form of cancer. Come to the surgery in future.'

'Oh, but doctor, that's awful harsh. You don't know what it's like. I pray every night for the Good Lord to take me.'

A weary sigh from the doctor.

'So do we, Mrs. Poole'

The 1990s saw the beginning of the AIDS epidemic. Some sufferers, British nationals living in the USA, found that their funds were dwindling, and insurance costs prohibitive, so they returned to Britain to seek further treatment, or, as often happened, terminal care. One such patient returned to our town, to spend his remaining months with his elderly mother. We offered him the best care available at the time, but he finally succumbed.

A GP from the practice called in on the mother to do a bereavement visit – to offer sympathy and to answer any questions.

'I'm mainly worried about his bed, doctor. I was thinking perhaps I would take it out into the back garden and burn it.'

'Oh, I don't think there's any need for that.' Then a pause that was a second too long.

'But I wouldn't sleep in it.'

I am at the on-call centre one evening, and my colleague is on the phone to a patient requesting a visit.

'I'm sorry, but home visits are restricted to those who can't make it to the out-of-hours centre.'

'You haven't got a car? Well, perhaps you can get someone to bring you in?'

'You don't know anyone who's got a car? Family, friends?'

'You haven't got any friends?'

'Well, you could always get a taxi.'

'I see, you can't walk to your front gate.'

'So, how did you get to the phone?'

A colleague from Kent tells the tale about a young lady who came to see him with a rather embarrassing problem. She had developed a dangly wart on her vulva. It was not only rather unsightly, but it got in the way of intimate encounters. My friend offered to remove it for her using cautery (think soldering iron). On the appointed day, she arrived at the surgery, was positioned on the couch, and the procedure began. Her nether regions were covered in a paper drape to preserve her dignity, some local anaesthetic was injected into the base of the wart, and the offending thing was removed easily using the cautery needle. Unfortunately, as my friend withdrew the hot needle, it touched the edge of the paper drape, which ignited. A minor conflagration ensued, but was quickly put out before any serious burns could occur. There was, however, shall we say, some deforestation in the Brazilian region.

Diabetes

It is impossible to be an expert in all things. So, inevitably, there will be some gaps in the encyclopaedia of medical knowledge for most practitioners. For me, it was diabetes. As an undergraduate, it had always been a bit of a mystery, and thankfully, it did not feature prominently in my finals. As a hospital doctor, I usually managed to recruit an expert opinion if the need arose. But now I was in general practice, where about 10% of my patient population would have this condition.

Shortly after starting in the job, I tentatively asked about the care of the diabetic population.

'They all go to the hospital diabetes clinic.' I was informed.

I quietly breathed a sigh of relief.

But it was not the case. I kept coming across diabetics who did not appear to have any sort of supervision. When I asked them why they were not going to the hospital clinic, I received some alarming responses.

'I don't like going there, they always tell me off.'

'I don't like the doctor, he's a darkie.'

'They don't even look at my results.'

'So, who is looking after your diabetes?'

'You are, doc.'

I decided that it was time for action. I arranged to see the consultant diabetologist, a charming, well-spoken Asian man with a shock of white hair styled into a quiff. I explained that, by my reckoning, about a third of my diabetic patients were receiving no formal care whatsoever.

'Well, why don't they come to the clinic?'

'They feel as they are being told off all the time,' I offered.

'Anything else?'

'Well, yes.' I cleared my throat. 'Some don't like you because you are a darkie.'

I anticipated rage, or at least, disgruntlement. Instead, he roared with laughter.

'Well, I can't change that, but we can change the system.'

We set up what was, in effect, a shared care system, so that all patients were under joint care. We communicated all findings, measurements, blood tests, so that no-one slipped through the net. He mentored me in diabetes care, building up my confidence. The system worked, and other practices started to take an interest. One day, he handed me a flyer, advertising a diabetes conference in London.

'I think you should go,' he said.

'Not sure if I can get the time off.'

'You really should go,' he persisted 'there are some excellent speakers.'

I scanned through the leaflet, and found to my horror that I was one of the excellent speakers.

And so it came to pass, that two months later, I stood on the stage of the Central Methodist Hall in Westminster, and nervously gave my first lecture. I had taken anti-diarrhoea tablets, and my tremor was barely noticeable from the back of the arena.

Further requests to speak followed, and I found myself immersed in the diabetes circus. I met the great and the good, and was invited to be a founding member of a fledgling national diabetes group called Primary Care Diabetes. This was a huge success, and eventually it morphed in to the Primary Care Diabetes Society, the largest primary care interest group in Europe. Over the next 25 years, I was to become involved in the launch of two prestigious journals, I wrote and edited books on diabetes and published several papers. I became chairman of a group called Primary Care Diabetes Europe.

But what was the most interesting was my involvement with the diabetes pharmaceutical industry. GPs who lecture are fairly rare. GPs who understand diabetes and lecture are even rarer. I was feted by the industry. I travelled widely, often business class, stayed in the best hotels, and was paid disproportionately high fees. My ego knew no bounds, but slowly, insidiously, I was being sucked into the murky world of big pharma. Of course, I believed everything the drug manufacturers said. I absorbed all the data from drug trials without questioning its real worth. I became so closely aligned with one or two companies that people thought I worked for them. My impartiality was often questioned, but I batted away any criticisms.

Then, one day, it all came crashing down around my ears. A major diabetes trial appeared to show that people taking one particular diabetes medication were more likely to suffer from cardiovascular disease. There were allegations that the pharmaceutical company who made the drug may have known about the problem from earlier, unpublished trials. The scales fell from my eyes. I began to see things in a different light. I questioned every finding of every trial. I refused to offer any endorsements, and I was extremely careful about being seen to support any one particular company.

What I learned was that the pharmaceutical companies are ultimately responsible to their shareholders, not to the people who take their products. This can lead to distortion of trial findings, suppression of negative trials, and misrepresentation of data.

Ben Goldacre, in his excellent book, Bad *Pharma* (Fourth Estate, Harper Collins, 2012), opens with a simple, but shocking, statement.

'Drugs are tested by the people who manufacture them, in poorly designed trials, on hopelessly small numbers of weird, unrepresentative patients, and analysed using techniques which are flawed by design, in such a way that they exaggerate the benefits of treatments.'

Wow. But he goes on to defend his statement, using multiple examples and clear logic. As I read each page, I found myself flushing with embarrassment, and the realisation that I had been a willing pawn in a rather seedy game. I had learned my lesson, perhaps a little too late. My final years in the realm of diabetes were tinged with guilt, but also a determination to encourage my colleagues to carefully examine every claim made by this industry.

Acts of sedition

I suppose there is a little bit of a rebel in all of us.

At school, there was the time when three of us decided to make a bomb in the chemistry lab. We had assembled the necessary ingredients in a crucible, inserted the electrodes, then retreated a safe distance before flicking the switch. There was a satisfying explosion, as the crucible shattered. A mushroom cloud of smoke rose from the bench as the chemistry teacher entered the lab. We expected a severe punishment, but he was actually very impressed, and even helped us to clean up the broken pieces.

Then there was the incident of the purple snow. A small canister, some potassium permanganate, a fuse, and hey presto! A twenty foot circle of purple snow.

I also got into trouble, in sixth form, for circulating a copy of The *Thoughts of Chairman Mao* which I had obtained during a visit to Lancaster University. And for writing a less-than-flattering poem about the French teacher, which I had foolishly left in my homework book.

At medical school, I kept my nose clean, ever fearful of providing an excuse for being expelled.

But, several years into my general practice career, an opportunity presented itself for the return to mischievous ways. Our director of public health at the time was very fond of producing strategy documents. A stop-smoking strategy was followed by a stroke strategy, a clean water strategy, and more, each delivered in an expensively bound document circulated to all GPs. I produced a spoof newsletter, outlining the need for a strategy to reduce strategies. This was illustrated with graphs and charts, and it was circulated widely, if anonymously. It was an instant hit. Emboldened by its success, I went on to produce spoof newspapers, targeting health management, specific consultants, the government. *Commissioning Weakly* was followed by *Symbiosis Monthly* (after a letter from the Health Trust that suggested that the NHS should be working in *symbiosis* with private providers).

This activity continued for some years, until an injudicious fax gave away the location of the miscreant, as it was easy to trace the number back to my surgery. There were no repercussions, other than furtive enquiries about when the next edition could be expected.

(Incidentally, I found myself one day, in the company of the aforementioned director of public health, in a seminar on *Determinants of Health*, a rather highbrow affair, looking at the factors which might influence the future health of our local population. We were all asked to call out the determinants which we felt would be crucial. 'Smoking status' said one. 'Poverty levels' called another. 'Nutritional status', 'employment', 'pollution' all followed. Then the director confidently added his contribution. 'Postcode' he said. There was an embarrassed silence, a few sniggers, and the chairman thankfully moved on. *Postcode? What on earth was he on about?* It is 2019, and access to simple investigations like x-rays, scans and ultrasound varies dramatically according to where you live in the UK. There are wide regional differences in services like physiotherapy, psychotherapy, even palliative care. So, I owe you a belated apology, director K.)

Here are some snippets from those publications;

SPY

Pleased to meet you, I'm a government spy
I'm trained to watch you, to just keep an eye
I know where you live, your date of birth
Your telephone number, and even your girth
I know who you sleep with, your sexual fears,
The number of partners you've had through the years.
The things that you smoke, be it Benson's or hash
The treatment you had for that strange little rash.
I know things that you have a yearning to hide
The seam of madness on your grandfather's side
The close acquaintance you had with the Bill

An unsavoury incident in Notting Hill
I know all your secrets, I've locked them away
You think that they're safe – they are, in a way
Nothing would tempt me to break that old vow
But for just a few quid, you may well allow
These delicate items to fall into the hand
Of people whose motives are not as you planned
When you sign on the line, be sure I will tell
Those intimate details, be sure I will sell
Your secrets, your data, your story, your life
And not just your own, but those of your wife
All with your permission to the highest bidders
From Norwich Union and Scottish Widders.
You fascinate other agencies too
My government friends – they care about you
They'd love all your data – if only they could
Like CCTV, it's for your own good
You know they have the noblest intentions
In planning your health, and trimming your pensions
Fear not, your life is not compromised
Computer data is anonymised
But birthdate and postcode, in the wrong hands
Will find you more swiftly than DNA strands
Don't misunderstand, I can be of use
Absolute power is prone to abuse
If you need a new fridge, or even a shower
I'll get it for you, I do have that power
You'd like a new flat in a nicer location
I'll do my best - that's my vocation
I alone pronounce you dead or alive
You're unfit to work, you're unfit to drive
Your benefits - they could go at a stroke
Your children, too – I'm afraid it's no joke
I'm in control from the womb to the tomb
And the funny thing is, as you sit in this room
You're quite unaware of the things I've discussed
In uncertain times it's me that you trust

So if that's all you need, I'll just see you later
I've got what I need, I've captured your data
Pleased to meet you, I'm a government spy
Here's your prescription. Goodbye.

(my wife thought I'd gone too far with that one.)

TEENAGE LAMENT

'E's burnin' up doctor
'E soaked all 'is beddin'
'E frew up in the night
It's doin' me 'ead in

'Is father could help me
If 'e wasn't in Reading
The prison I mean
And it's doin' me 'ead in

'E started on cider
Then moved on to dope
Then on to 'eroin
And me I can't cope

I 'spect it's a virus
'E's bin sick on 'is vest
I ain't got no calpol
And I'm really depressed

'E won't take 'is feeds, yeah
I just give up 'ope
I ain't got no calpol
And me I can't cope

121

I went down the social
They wasn't impressed
I cashed in me Giro
But I'm really depressed

I goes out wiv me mates right
We 'ad vodka and lime
I frew up in the taxi
And I'm tired all the time

I went round me nan's yeah
She sez not to mope
She's got Parkinson's whatsname
Well me, I can't cope

They sent me a letter
You'd fink it's a crime
'e ain't 'ad 'is jabs yet
And I'm tired all the time

'E's good as gold really
I'm doin' me best
I've got massive 'eadache
And I'm really depressed

I'm sixteen next Sat'day
I'm plannin' me weddin'
Well after this next kid
It's doin' me 'ead in

DISCHARGE SUMMARY FIASCO

The Primary Healthcare Trust has this week apologised to a local GP for the early arrival of a discharge summary relating to a 63 year old man. The patient, admitted for routine surgery, was discharged in August. The discharge letter apparently arrived within a week. A trust spokesman said 'We apologise for this oversight. It contravenes our policy of waiting at least a year before sending out the letter. I understand the discharge summary contained useful information and an updated medication list. I am devastated that this has happened.' The GP, who does not wish to be named, was clearly appalled. 'Sending out discharge summaries this early is indecent. We need the academic challenge of trying to piece together what happened to the patient over a period of months.'

'SUPERBUG' SHOCK

A local woman was said to be 'shocked but comfortable' last night after failing to contract a 'superbug' infection following routine surgery at a local hospital. The woman, in her late forties, told *Symbiosis Weekly* 'It all seemed to be so straightforward, but two days after the operation, doctors broke the news to me. I mean you read about these things in the papers but you never think it could happen to you.' Last night she was being comforted by relatives. It is thought that there have been three other similar cases this year.

'FAT-CAT GP' DENIAL

Press reports that GPs are working fewer hours for hugely inflated salaries are 'unfounded and inflammatory' an enraged GP claimed today. Speaking after the careful examination of a divot on the 14th fairway, the doctor opined 'The people who write these sorts of reports are unaware of the vast increase in paperwork that accompanies modern general practice. In addition to repeat prescriptions, there are holiday booking forms, share applications, premium bond certificates and new car warranties to cope with.' Challenged about reports that 50% of GPs earn over £200,000 per year, he angrily retorted 'That's preposterous! I imagine the exact opposite is true – 50% of GPs **don't** earn over £200,000 per year.'

Complaints

When I qualified in general practice, complaints against GPs were very rare. Perhaps, on reflection, too rare. If a loved one died in your care it was a case of 'well, you did your best for him, doctor.' If mistakes occurred, then it was 'well, these things happen, don't they?' Patients were grateful for anything you did, and doctors had a sort of God-like status, imperious, beyond criticism. That has all changed, thanks to the compensation culture we are now saddled with. Biased reporting in the national press, sensationalist headlines in magazines, all telling you that you must complain, you have rights, this sort of thing shouldn't happen. Even the ambulance chasing packs of solicitors have moved on from 'Have you been in an accident that wasn't your fault?' to 'Did your GP make an incorrect or late diagnosis?' The implication is that an apology is not enough, there must be money in it somewhere. Of course, there does have to be accountability, and the profession has strict rules and guidelines about behaviour and competency. But it has gone too far, and the fear of medicolegal proceedings casts a cloud over the profession, and may be a factor in the headlong rush towards early retirement.

I was in my first year of practice when a young lad presented with tummyache. He looked ill, and my examination confirmed my suspicion that he had acute appendicitis. I turned to his father and said 'He needs to be in hospital', whereupon the young patient burst into tears. I laid a comforting hand on his head, and said 'never mind, you'll get a couple of weeks off school.' He was admitted to hospital, the offending appendix was duly removed, and he made a full recovery. Shortly afterwards, my senior partner came to see me, an embarrassed look on his face. He perched awkwardly on the corner of my desk, and told me that there had been a complaint. The father of the small boy had reported that I claimed that he was making his symptoms up to get time off school. The senior partner suggested that I should apologise.

'If he wants to talk to me about this, he can come and see me personally,' was my reply.

To his credit, he did come and see me. I went through the details of the case with him.

'Did I listen to the account of his symptoms?' Yes.

'Did I carefully examine him.' Yes.

'Did I make the correct diagnosis, and send him to hospital?' Yes.

'Did I comfort him when he was upset?' Yes.

'Is he now making a full recovery?' Yes.

'Well, what precisely are you doing here?'

He had the good grace to apologise himself for making such an unwarranted fuss.

Move on thirty years. As the senior partner, I am in charge of any complaints that arise in the practice. Due to the shift described above, these are more frequent. Often trivial, often irrelevant to the practice – 'I can't get an appointment with the orthopaedic surgeon for three months' – not my fault. Most complaints are dealt with swiftly and easily, an apology for a rude receptionist, an apology for an item missed off a repeat prescription.

One morning, the practice manager arrives in my office, looking uncharacteristically flustered.

'There's been a complaint.'

I roll my eyes. 'Who is it this time?' I ask, with a sigh.

'Well, it's.....it's about you.'

'Oh.'

'Do you remember seeing a small child in surgery this morning with abdominal pain?'

I do remember, and suddenly my mind is spinning, running rapidly through the consultation. He had abdominal pain, I examined him,

126

thought it was just a normal tummyache, nothing serious, take some Calpol, day off school.

'Oh God, I didn't miss something, did I?'

'No, it's not about that, but did you make any reference to the colour of his hair?'

Another replay. Worried mum, worried child, ruffle his hair in a friendly way...

'Don't worry........carrot top.'

His mother had taken exception to this little phrase of endearment. I was forced to make a grovelling apology to her.

I returned home that evening and replayed the whole incident to my wife. I had hoped for sympathy and understanding, a glass of wine, a comforting hug. She was incandescent.

'YOU SAID WHAT?'

She then lectured me on the exquisite sensitivity pertaining to people of a ginger persuasion. I was about to mention that he was ugly as well, but thought better of it.

A few weeks later, we were visiting our son in Brighton. Strolling along the promenade, we bumped into his boss, who was pushing a pram containing their new offspring. He turned the pram round to proudly display his son, sporting a shock of, shall we say, reddish hair. My wife and my son both looked at me, horror struck and filled with dreadful anticipation. Out of the line of sight of his boss, my son drew a finger across his throat. I got the message.

'Aaah' I cooed, 'hasn't he got lovely......(savouring the moment)...eyes.'

An ordinary day

It is Saturday afternoon, and I am on call for the practice. The workload is steadily building, bringing with it the usual litany of coughs, rashes, bellyache. The bleep goes off. A temporary resident, called Mr. Theodopolous, is staying at a hotel on the seafront. He has swollen ankles. 'I'll get round to him when I can', I tell the family, it's rather busy right now'. The bleep goes off again. 'It's a young girl, pregnant, thinks she might be in labour, but her boyfriend is threatening to stamp on the baby when it comes out.' Well, that's different. I recognise the address, and recall that one of the residents, a large, scruffy, menacing man, has serious mental health issues, which, up to this point, had been fairly well controlled with medication. I immediately visit to assess the situation. It is pretty much as I feared, things are tense, and I don't think a stern talking-to will do the trick. I call the duty social worker, and the duty psychiatrist, as I am in no doubt that we are going to have to 'section' the patient under the Mental Health Act. The psychiatrist suggests we have police backup in case things turn even nastier. The bleep goes again - Mr. Theodopolous, wondering how long I'll be. 'I'm a bit tied up right now, it might be some time'.

Once the police, social services, and the psychiatrist have co-ordinated their arrival, we enter the house clutching our forms. It is the duty of the social worker to ensure fair play, in effect, protecting the interests of the patient, and ensuring we are not misusing our powers under the Mental Health Act. The psychiatrist is there to assess the current mental condition of the patient. The police are there to maintain order. I am there to make up the numbers and sign the forms. Things, predictably, do take a turn for the worse. The threatening boyfriend is in no mood for compromise. The baby is the child of the devil, and needs to be killed. We are all agreed, the forms are signed, and the baby-stamper is carted off.

The bleep goes off again. Elderly lady, thinks she might have coughed up some blood. I arrive to find a very thin, very pale lady who really does not want to bother me on a Saturday. I take her history and examine her. She has been losing weight for some time, her appetite is poor, partly because, she explains, she has had difficulty swallowing. On examination, she is deathly pale, and has clearly lost more than 'a bit of weight.' I ask her if she has kept any of the blood she coughed up. She leads me to the bathroom, where I find a blood soaked towel in the bath, containing at least two pints of blood. She clearly has got cancer of the oesophagus, and is at risk of perforating, with probably fatal consequences. I arrange an urgent ambulance. Whilst I am on the phone, ambulance control, who also operate the bleep system, mention that Mr. Theodopolous has rung twice more.

What on earth is the matter with the man? It's just swollen ankles. Given all that I have had to endure today, it's hardly that urgent. I catch up on my other calls, dispensing antibiotics, advice and good cheer in equal amounts. Eventually, late afternoon, I arrive at the Golden Bay Hotel. Mr. Theodopolous is lying on the bed, surrounded by anxious family members. I try to suppress my exasperation, dearly wanting to shout out 'Do you know what sort of day I've had?' My professionalism takes over, and I peel back the sheets to take a closer look at the famed swollen ankles. The swelling goes from his almost unrecognisable feet, up his tree-trunk sized legs, into his groin, where his testicles have taken on elephantine proportions. I peer at his less than Mediterranean colouring. He is not so much olive-skinned as the colour of light olive oil.

'Can you tell me a little about his medical history?' I venture.

'Well, doctor, he does have a blood problem.'

The penny drops. Or the drachma. Greek chap, blood disorder, swollen legs. Any third year medical student would be screaming in my ear by now. The swollen legs are due to advanced heart failure, caused in turn by extreme anaemia.

'This blood disorder, it wouldn't by any chance be thalassaemia, would it?'

'That's the one, doctor.'

Thalassaemia is a rare inherited blood disorder, common in Mediterranean races, characterised by anaemia (thinning of the blood). I admit him to hospital, and the incredibly enthusiastic house officer later rings me to tell me that Mr. Theodopolous had a haemoglobin level of 4 on admission. The normal level is about 15.

'How was your day?' asks my wife when I eventually return home.

'Oh, you know, just the usual.'

Out with the old – the new GP contract

Those of us who worked in general practice in the 1980s and 1990s had become inured to the intransigence of the government in relation to the future of the profession. We had heard the false promises, endured pay freezes, experienced poor working conditions, and the lack of investment in premises. However, towards the end of the 1990s, things started to turn sour. A new breed of GP was emerging, tougher, smarter, more militant. There was talk of strikes, even mass resignations. Eventually, after protracted negotiations, the new GP contract was agreed and it came in to force on April 1st 2004. This promised a better pay deal, and improved working conditions

Perhaps the most exciting development was the chance to 'opt out' of the out-of-hours commitment. Since the inception of the NHS, GPs had been required to provide 24-hour cover for their patients. Now, we had a choice. Here, as in many other things, the government had underestimated the will and determination of GPs. This 'opt out' came at a price. It would cost an individual GP £6000 per year. £6000? Are you serious? After years of working antisocial hours and weekends. The vast majority of GPs decided it was worth a measly £6000 to have a much better quality of life. In our area, ALL the GPs went for it. This posed some problems for the new Primary Care Trust.

'Ah, we see that you have all opted out.'

'Yep.'

'Only......who is going to look after the patients after 6.30 p.m?'

'Well, the new contract says it is your responsibility.'

'But....we have no doctors.'

The equivalent of a mass Gallic shrug.

'Of course, we *could* do the on-call for you....'

'Go on...' (excitedly)

'But it wouldn't be for nothing, as in the bad old days, we would want a commercially viable rate.'

'How much?'

'££££'

'How much?'

'Take it or leave it.'

And so it was that GP co-operatives sprang up, and GPs were paid a fortune for their efforts.

The old contract paid General Practitioners (GPs) on the basis of fees and allowances. In contrast, the new contract allocated resources to GPs through three main funding streams: the global sum; the Quality and Outcomes Framework (QOF); and enhanced services payments. Separate funding streams were available for practices to modernise their premises and improve their IT infrastructure.

The global sum was a big chunk of money to cover the nuts and bolts of running a practice. The QOF (more of this later) was a controversial system of paying GPs for collection points, based on set quality standards. Enhanced services covered such things as minor operations, immunisations and so on. As the global sum was pretty much a guess, there was an amount called the MPIG – Minimum Practice Income Guarantee – in case they got it wildly wrong. This was added to the global sum.

Bearing in mind that the new contract represented the single biggest change in the profession since 1948, we had received amazingly little information in the months leading up to the date when we had to sign on the dotted line. A meeting eventually took place between the new paymasters, the Primary Care Trust (PCT) and the partners in the practice, in March 2014, once month before the start date. I took detailed notes during that meeting, and wrote up my notes immediately afterwards. The following account is an accurate, (almost verbatim) record. It may read like a comedy script, but it generated few laughs at the time.

PCT: We are here today to discuss the implications of the new GMS contract, which will represent, in effect, the greatest change in the delivery of primary care services since the inception of the MHS. We will outline the impact it will have on your practice, its organisation, and its income.

US: But we haven't seen the final version of the contract yet.

PCT: It will be out soon.

US: How long is it?

PCT: 320 pages.

US: And if we decide not to sign it?

PCT: Then you can sign the default contract.

US: What does that look like?

PCT: It will be out soon.

US: So, let's get this straight. You want us to sign a contract we haven't seen, based on figures we haven't received, or choose an alternate contract, which we also haven't seen?

PCT: Ah, but we do have some figure for you, and after all, you still have a month to decide.

US: Let's see those figures.

PCT: This is your global sum.

US: It doesn't look very big.

PCT: Don't worry, that's not the final figure.

US: When will we have the final figure?

PCT: We'' have a better idea in April.

US: After we've signed?

PCT: Yes, but don't worry about that – look at the global sum.

US: It still doesn't look very big.

PCT: Ah, yes, but that doesn't take into consideration the MPIG.

US: The MPIG?

PCT: The Minimum Practice Income Guarantee. It's a sum of money which the government has allocated in the exceptional circumstance that we get your global sum wrong.

US: And how many practices in this area get this MPIG?

PCT: They all do.

US: So you got all the global sums wrong?

PCT: They're provisional.

US: What are these figures based on?

PCT: Well, partly on your list size, shown here.

US: That's not our list size.

PCT: Isn't it? It was two years ago.

US: It's gone up 600 since then.

PCT: Well, it's near enough for now. And anyway, we also have to consider enhanced services.

US: Such as?

PCT: Well, minor operations.

US: How much will we be paid for those?

PCT: We can't tell you.

US: You can tell us, we're doctors.

PCT: Well, it all depends.

US: On what?

PCT: On how many you do.

US: That will depend on how much we get paid.

PCT: Well you won't do too many. Will you?

US: Why?

PCT: Because we haven't got a lot of money. So what we've decided to do is not to pay you for the first few months, see how many you do, then decide how much of the money to give you.

US: What about minor injuries?

PCT: Oh yes – we have a sum set aside for that.

US: And how much will we get?

PCT: We can't tell you.

US: You can tell us, we're doctors.

PCT: Well, it depends how much you do.

US: That depends on how much we get.

PCT: Well, shall we just leave it that we won't give you anything to start with, and see how things go?

US: This is becoming a recurrent theme.

PCT: Let's move on to Quality and Outcome payments.

US: We WILL get paid those, won't we?

PCT: OF course. You get one third of the money as an aspiration payment, and the rest as a reward payment.

US: At the end of the year?

PCT: Well, it will technically be the end of the year, but you won't get paid until April.

US: That's the next year.

PCT: Yes, but it will be included in your March figures, so it will feel like you've been paid that year.

US: And how much will that be?

PCT: £75 per point, adjusted according to a practice factor, then adjusted according to the prevalence formula.

US: What prevalence formula?

PCT: The prevalence of the illnesses included in the framework.

US: What is the prevalence?

PCT: We don't know.

US: When will you know?

PCT: On National Prevalence Day.

136

US: When's that?

PCT: Next February.

US: So, at present, it is not possible to calculate this element of our income?

PCT: No, but don't let that deter you from signing the contract. Oh, and we forgot to mention the April payment.

US: What about it?

PCT: Well, it might be smaller than you are expecting, as it won't include many of the things you now get paid for, and it also won't include many of the things you might get paid for, but we don't know how much, and the things you will get paid for, but we don't know how much.

US: Why are you telling us this?

PCT: So you will have time to arrange a loan to cover your practice expenses.

US: And you'll pay the interest?

PCT: No, it's nothing to do with us.

US: I thought the new contract promised us all a 50% pay rise.

PCT: We believe you will feel it coming through.

US: Well, at least, under the new contract, we could close our list if things get too much for us.

PCT: I wouldn't do that.

US: Why not?

PCT: It would send out the wrong message.

US: How do you mean?

PCT: We might think that you didn't feel able to take on the enhanced services we will be paying you for, once we know how much you will be doing, and therefore how much to pay you.

US: On the contrary, it might mean that we have decided to concentrate our efforts on providing high quality services to a defined population.

PCT: We wouldn't see it like that.

US: So you would prefer us to keep our list open, and risk providing a progressively poorer quality service to an increasingly larger population?

PCT: Anyway, it's time to go. We hope this meeting has been helpful and informative, and allayed any fears you might have had about signing the contract.

US: Well, let's recap. We are expected to sign a contract we haven't seen, which is offering a global sum which is less than we had two years ago, topped up by aMPIG based on an out of date practice list size, supplemented by various unknown sums of money, and a quality payment based on a formula which won't be calculated until next year. If we decline, we can sign a default contract we haven't yet seen. If we accept, our initial income will plunge us into debt, and neither we nor you have the faintest idea how much we stand to earn over the next two years?

PCT: We wouldn't see it like that. We prefer to think of it as *'The modern, dependable NHS'*.

US: We'll let you know.

We signed the contract on 30th March 2004.

QOF – the Quality and Outcomes Framework

'Twas the ever-rambunctious Ken Clarke, then Secretary of state for Health who is credited with saying 'whenever there is talk of change, you will find general practitioners reaching nervously for their wallets.' Harsh, you might think, but undeniably true. It is a popular misconception that GPs are salaried by the NHS. They are not. They are self-employed individuals who contract their services to the NHS. This came about at the inception of the NHS, and has been the case ever since, though successive governments have tried, and failed, to change it.

So, each practice is, in effect, a business. There are streams of income, there are expenses, and there are profits. The profits are what line our pockets when all is taken care of. Therefore, each NHS change or re-organisation leads us to focus on the implications, and to develop a strategy to maintain our income, whilst at the same time maintaining high standards, and delivering a high quality service.

As part of the new contract, we saw the introduction of the Quality and Outcomes Framework, which became known simply as QOF (pronounced 'quaff', not 'cough'). This was a system of payments for performance, or quality, as the government at the time defined it. Put simply, in its first incarnation, there were 1000 points on offer, each with money attached, for the attainment of various targets. These were divided into disease categories, such as asthma and diabetes. For example, at the time, there were 100 points for diabetes, which 'encouraged' GPs to hit targets for blood pressure measurement, smoking cessation, eye checks, kidney tests, and so on. All very laudable, but full of holes and inconsistencies.

But, to paraphrase that game-show jingle 'points mean prizes.' The government assumed that the introduction of the QOF would cause some organisational problems for GPs, that they would take some time to adjust to the new system. And so they budgeted for a maximum attainment of 750 points out of a possible 1000.

WRONG! They should have listened to good ol' Ken Clarke. Their income was at stake. If there were 1000 points on offer, they were going to get 1000 points, no matter what organisational change was needed. Clinics were set up, nurses recruited, QOF staff recruited, computer programs installed. At the end of year one, the average attainment was about 950 points per practice. 'Ah', the government said, 'there is a problem. You have done too well.'

Too well?? What, we have provided too much quality? Yes, we had, and there would be a clawback, a penalty for over performing. Can you imagine this principle applying to, for example, the business community? 'Your bank has been too successful, you'll have to pay for it.' Or education – 'your results are too good, too many A grades at A-level, there'll be hell to pay for this.'

I was opposed to QOF from the start, and made my position clear. I wrote a piece for one of the GP newspapers. This was picked up by The Independent, and they sent a reporter to interview me. I had made the point that conditions covered by the QOF, and which generated income, would take precedence, and that other conditions, such as arthritis and Parkinson's disease, would become neglected, as resources would be concentrated elsewhere. Scandalous? No, far from it. This proved to be quite accurate, and led to lobbying from patient groups for specific conditions, such as Alzheimer's disease, to be included in the QOF.

But one of my main objections about QOF was that it encouraged devious means of fiddling the data. For example, one of the targets related to the management of depression. Certain procedures had to be followed, in a person newly diagnosed with this condition, in order to get the points. But if it looked like you were going to miss 'the target', you could enter a diagnosis of 'low mood' instead, thereby escaping the net. There were other examples of alternative diagnostic codes being used in this way. Does it matter? Well. Yes it does. The United Kingdom has one of the best, if not the best, data collection systems in the world. These data are used for research and statistical purposes, and it behoves us to maintain strict levels of accuracy.

There was also the 'March effect'. QOF data were collected and collated at the end of March. So, if you had reached the necessary targets, there was no call to panic. For example, if enough patients had hit the blood pressure targets, why rock the boat? So, blood pressure checks scheduled for March could be moved forward to April, lest some readings had gone up and ruined your figures. Conversely, a diabetic with raised blood sugar readings might find that their medication was increased before March in order for them to duck under the necessary line in time.

QOF underwent many modifications over subsequent years, but it is still in existence today, apart from in Wales, where it was abandoned, in an attempt to attract GPs in to a land whose primary care was in terminal decline, with hundreds of unfilled GP posts.

Skiing

Both James and I were keen skiers. Every year, we would take ourselves off to the slopes, usually as part of a larger group. One regular attendee was a larger-than-life Welshman called Colin. He became famous as much for his off-piste activities as for his heroic attempts on the white stuff.

One day, we found him sprawled on the snow, wincing painfully. He had strayed unintentionally off-piste, and collided with a ski-lift stanchion. He pointed to his foot.

'Tell you what, boy, this is giving a bit of gip.'

We removed his ski boot and sock, and found that he had a rapidly developing sub-ungual haematoma. This is a bleed underneath the toenail. As the blood can't escape, it pushes steadily against the nail, causing considerable pain. The solution is to release the blood. In the confines of the surgery, this would be done with a hot wire or diathermy needle. Anaesthetic is not required, as the nail has no feeling, and it is now separated from the sensitive nail bed by a lake of high pressure blood. James decided to improvise. He unscrewed the side of his sunglasses, heated it with a cigarette lighter and applied it to the nail. The result was an impressive fountain of blood, staining the surrounding snow a delightful shade of crimson, and a few Welsh expletives. Job done.

On another occasion, the hapless Colin was involved in a collision with a snowboarder. He was winded, but able to make it back to the chalet. That evening, he quietly approached me after dinner.

'Could you take a look at something?'

We disappeared into his room, where he bared all. The bruising from the earlier collision had spread across his lower abdomen, and had caused one testicle, and half his penis, to turn purple. I explained that this would settle over the next couple of weeks.

'Just worried how I was going to explain to the lads at the rugby club how I had developed a two-tone todger.' Needless to say, this was to become his nom-de-guerre.

Eating and drinking on the slopes can be a pricey affair. Colin had the answer. At breakfast time, he would surreptitiously squirrel away some rolls, some cheese, some ham. He would then make sandwiches for consumption later. As we met for lunch one day, he asked 'Just how waterproof do you think clingfilm is?' I gave a non-committal reply. 'I mean, is it really, really waterproof?' Pressed about this obsession, he revealed that, as his one-piece ski-suit had no pockets, he stuffed his wrapped sandwiches down the front. On a visit to the toilet, he had unzipped his outfit, and his lunch had fallen out and dropped into the toilet bowl.

'What did you do?' I asked, already dreading the response.

'You've got to believe in clingfilm, boyo', he announced as he proudly flourished the rolls, unwrapped and ate the (hopefully) preserved contents.

But the main reason for including these skiing anecdotes (apart from the sketchy medical content), is an encounter that occurred on a chair-lift. I found myself, as you often do, seated next to a stranger. He turned out to be English, from Surrey, and a fellow GP.

'So are you here with a group, or what?'

'Well, I've come with my partner.'

'Your wife?'

'No, my partner in the practice.'

He looked at me, incredulous.

'I can't imagine anything worse. I hate my partners, can't wait to get away from them for a week.'

'Well, it's not like that in my practice. We all quite like each other. We often all go out together for meals with our spouses.'

He shook his head. A silence followed, then a thought struck him.

'If you're here, and your partner is here, who is looking after the practice?'

'That's easy', I replied, 'the other partners come in and work on their days off, so that we can get away.'

He almost fell out of the ski-lift.

I realised that I was incredibly fortunate to work with kind, like-minded individuals, in a practice that valued quality of life more than the relentless quest for wealth. Supportive, reasonable, friends as well as partners, this cocooned life was my existence for over thirty years. I can hardly remember a cross word between us in all that time.

It's not that serious

I have been amazed about the lack of seriousness that some patients attach to their symptoms and conditions. It is not unusual for patients to turn up with a history of bleeding from their bowels, bladder, nose, eardrum, or other bodily parts. In response to the question 'How long has this been going on?', they offer 'just a few months'. 'Why haven't you come to see me sooner?' 'Didn't think it was anything serious.' What, then, dear patient, did you think it was? Normal??

John was a 56 year old programmer who worked for a financial institution in Bond Street, London. He commuted daily. He was a thin, non-smoking, non-drinking man who cycled a great deal and was physically fit. One day, he was sitting at his computer when he experienced central chest pain. 'It's probably a heart attack' he told himself. Computer programmers are almost by definition 'on the spectrum' i.e. wired differently from the rest of us. You or I might immediately dial 999 and demand an ambulance as soon as possible. John's logic was different. 'If I dial 999, the ambulance will take me to a local hospital, where it will be inconvenient for my friends and family to visit. Therefore, it is logical to return home at this point. The heart attack will not have had the chance to develop to a critical point yet.' Unbelievably, he travelled across London and boarded a train for the 90 minute journey home. He rang his wife, with an interesting twist on the usual 'I'm on the train' conversation.

'Hello, darling, I'm on the train, and I'm having a heart attack. Can you pick me up at the station and take me to the hospital?'

His furious wife did exactly what was asked. The receiving doctor at A and E immediately arranged an ECG which showed a myocardial infarction (posh for heart attack), he was seen by the cardiologist, transferred to intensive care, and had a stent fitted within the hour. He made a full recovery.

Another patient who arrived at the surgery in the middle of a heart attack absconded from the treatment room as the ambulance was on its way, got into his car, and drove to the hospital himself, on the grounds that his car was on a parking meter.

Martin was a well respected teacher in his 40s when I first made his acquaintance. His wife had a good job in an administrative role. As was not uncommon in a small town, they were on the fringes of our social circuit, as well as being patients of the practice. Martin enjoyed the occasional glass of red wine, so much so, that at some social events, he would pass out before the end of the evening. His wife would try to cover for him by explaining that Martin was 'stressed and tired'. There is a wealth of difference between stifling a yawn, and being face down in your dessert next to an empty wine bottle. Over the years, the situation became worse. When he attended the surgery for an unrelated problem, I took the opportunity to check his liver function tests. Unsurprisingly, they came back with abnormalities. I called him in to the surgery, sat him down and politely, but firmly, suggested that he needed to do something about his drinking. 'But I do like a glass of red wine,' was the innocent reply. Gradually things deteriorated, both medically and socially. One morning, he was stopped by the police on the way to work, and was found to be over the limit from the previous night's drinking. He lost his job, and shortly afterwards, his wife left him. His liver disease progressed to the point that he was referred to a liver specialist. He told him firmly, and not so politely, to stop drinking. Forever. Full stop. He came to see me in the surgery, complaining that his skin and his eyes were turning yellow. 'Martin, it's your liver, its packing up, the yellow skin is jaundice due to advanced liver disease. You must stop drinking completely'. 'But I just like a glass of red wine'. I was becoming exasperated. 'You don't get it, do you? You have lost your job, your wife, your house, your health, and you are about to lose your life.' 'Well, how about a glass just every other night?' He died some months later, presumably still thinking he did not have a serious problem.

Is there a doctor in the house?

It is inevitable that, at some point in your professional career, you will be called upon to render your expert medical services in a setting other than your practice or the hospital setting. These days, this is more likely to occur on a plane journey, rather than the 'house' setting of a theatre. Of course, you respond positively to the request, as it behoves you to have a duty of care to your fellow man, woman or child. There is always a degree of trepidation, caused both by the thought of performing in the public arena, and also of the risk of getting something wrong. The prospect of litigation, when you are simply doing your best, is very real indeed. So much so that a 'good Samaritan' clause had to be introduced in the USA, amongst other places, as medical professionals were refusing to intervene in such circumstances, lest they were subject to a law suit.

Anyway, whenever the situation does arise, it is almost always the rule that, when you get to the person at the centre of the medical emergency, another, probably more highly qualified health professional will get there first. I was strolling along the seafront one sunny day, when I became aware of a kerfuffle up ahead. A man lay collapsed on the pavement, surrounded by a small crowd. A quick glance confirmed that, in addition to a consultant surgeon, there were, in attendance, a theatre technician, a nurse, and an undertaker. Furthermore, the 'patient' was well known to me as someone who was prone to hysterical collapse i.e. falling on the ground, with no medical cause, and feigning unconsciousness, to gain attention. Thus reassured, I continued on my way.

On another occasion, I was travelling to New York when I was informed that a woman had collapsed outside the toilet at the rear of the plane. I made my way there, to be greeted by the sight of no less than five American cardiologists, who had been attending a conference. They seemed to have the situation under control, but I was at a loss to see how they would be able to render appropriate assistance without the tools of their trade – cash register, invoice book, and credit card machine.

More recently, I was returning from a holiday in Spain when the call went out. I raised my hand. The flight attendant asked 'Do you speak Spanish?' I replied in the negative, but got up to offer assistance. Apparently, a small boy had developed abdominal pain, and his father was convinced he had appendicitis. By the time I got there, a Spanish-speaking consultant paediatrician was in attendance. Bueno!

But the prize for best story has to go to my lovely wife, a trained nurse, who was on her way to work early one morning, when she came across a chap sitting on the pavement, leaning against a car. My wife quickly ascertained that he was, sadly, deceased. Very deceased. At that point in time, she was unceremoniously pushed out of the way by a frantic-looking woman.

'We need to start CPR!' she shouted.

'I'm afraid he's dead.'

'No, you don't understand, we need to start now.'

She laid a finger on his cold wrist, and convinced herself there was a pulse.

'There really isn't much point' explained my wife, 'he has been dead for some time.'

'No, YOU don't understand, *I work on the pharmacy counter in Boots!*'

Faced with such undeniable expertise, and as she was already late, my wife left her to it.

Doctor Who?

It goes with the job, being recognised in public places in the practice area. Walking round Tesco, I would encounter many patients, who would greet me cordially, whilst having one eye on the contents of my trolley. *Plenty of fruit and vegetables, some fish, but what's that? A Ginster's Cornish pasty? Two bottles of wine?*

The reverse situation would also commonly occur. I would pop in to the bank or post office, to be served by a young woman who had flushed to the roots of her hair, and I would rack my brains to remember just what embarrassing complaint she had presented with.

For the most part, these encounters were good natured, and it felt good to be respected as a pillar of the community. Sometimes, it was a bit intrusive, such as when you are out for a walk with the family, only to be hailed loudly by some bumptious character, shouting 'Hey, doc, that cream you gave me didn't work.'

But my fame also spread outside the practice area. On one occasion, I had taken the overnight ferry to Le Havre, and was having an early morning coffee on the quay at Honfleur, when a strolling passer-by said 'Morning, doc!'

I was also recognised as I sat on the snow in a little known French ski resort, having spectacularly fallen off the drag lift. 'You'll never learn to ski like tha,t doc.'

On a visit to some family in Lancashire, we had visited the set of *Coronation Street*. The following week, a patient presented me with a photo he had taken of me and my family outside the *Rover's Return*. 'Never thought I'd see you there, doc.'

On a cruise from Florida, we called in to the Cayman Islands. Trying to get our bearings, I asked a very British-looking bobby for directions. I detected an accent, and asked him where he was from. He had grown up in my practice area, and his parents were my patients.

And some of my youngest patients, who had misheard my name being called in the surgery, thought I was Doctor *Who*. I chose not to disavow them of this notion, and would delight in their open-mouthed astonishment if they saw me in the street, especially if I was wearing a long scarf.I=

THE DOCTOR. In those days, there was an unspoked respect for the professional, now sadly diminished. I might be on a late night call in a less salubrious part of the practice. My bag would contain controlled drugs and prescription pads – valuable items. I would approach a group of slouching, hoodie wearing youths, smoking and laughing.

'I'm THE DOCTOR. I'm looking for flat five.'

'Ok, doc, it's round the back, let me show you there.'

These days, I would be accompanied by the on-call driver, lest someone was tempted to pull out a knife. No timelord status now.

The Shipman Effect

Harold Frederick Shipman was a general practitioner in Hyde, Cheshire. On 31st January 2000, a jury found him guilty of the murders of 215 patients. He was sentenced to life imprisonment. He hanged himself in prison the day before his 58th birthday. He was one of the most prolific serial killers in history. He is the only British doctor to have been found guilty of murdering his patients, though others, including Bodkin Adams, have been suspected. He had his first position as a GP in Todmorden in Yorkshire. Whilst there, he was found guilty of forging prescriptions for pethidine for his own use. He was fined £600, attended a drug rehabilitation clinic, and was allowed to return to general practice. He moved to Hyde, where he became established as a respected member of the community. In 1998, a local GP and a local funeral parlour expressed concerns to the coroner about the high death rate among Dr Shipman's patients. The investigation was abandoned. Later in 1998, a local taxi driver contacted the police, informing them that he believed Shipman was killing his patients. He was eventually caught after forging the will of one of his victims, which left him £386,000.

The day that the story broke, I wrote to the editor of The Daily Telegraph suggesting that Shipman must have wanted to be caught, because he had been clever enough to conceal his crimes up until the unbelievably stupid error of the forgery. I went further than that. I suggested that it was possible, if not probable, that GPs up and down the country were 'helping' their patients to die, mostly for humane reasons, such as terminal illness and intractable pain. The letter was not published.

On 11th February 2000, 10 days after his conviction, the General Medical Council struck Shipman off the register!

The Shipman enquiry report, conducted by Dame Janet Smith, made several recommendations which led to changes in standard medical procedures in Britain. Other changes, which did not spring directly from this report, led to the so-called 'Shipman effect'. I shall describe some of the features of this effect, and tell you all why I think it has made not a jot of difference to the possibility of another Shipman, though probably less prolific, working in modern day general practice.

Death certificates and cremation.

If you are the sort of person who traces their ancestry, in the vague hope of finding some connection to royalty, you will have encountered parish records at some stage. You might find that one of your relatives died from 'consumption' (this does not mean that someone ate him – it is the old word for tuberculosis), or 'shaking palsy' – probably Parkinson's disease or some such. You might also encounter 'madness', or even 'worn out' given as the medical cause of death. Since then, things have changed. In my own early days, it was permissible to enter 'old age' as a cause of death. Nowadays, you need to be more specific. If Ethel dies in a nursing home aged 101, she of course died from 'cardiopulmonary degeneration' i.e. old age. The doctor cannot just put 'cancer', it needs to be 'cancer of the lung' for example. Similarly, 'septicaemia' needs to be 'septicaemia due to gangrene of the leg'. Leaving aside the semantic issues, there remains the question of accuracy. The certifying doctor can put down anything that is *reasonably accurate*, but there is a requirement that he or she has attended the patient in the fourteen days before death. So, if I see John Smith on 1st April, and he is complaining of a severe chest infection, and he dies on April 10th, it would be r*easonable* to state 'chest infection' or perhaps 'pneumonia' as the cause of death. The thing is, John Smith might have started to get chest pains on the 9th of April, putting it down to his chest condition, when actually is was the first sign of the heart attack that caused him to draw his last breath. We won't know, unless there is a post mortem, and that is not required as the doctor is acting within the law, and there are no suspicious circumstances. Returning to Harold Shipman, therefore, he certainly attended the deceased within fourteen days of their demise (usually within fourteen minutes, as he was the one wielding the large syringe filled with morphine), and as he had carefully written in the medical records 'complaining of chest pain', he was fully entitled to give the cause of death as 'coronary artery disease' or 'cardiac arrest' or 'pneumonia', and no-one would question it. But someone did – a local GP concerned about the numbers of Shipman's previously robust patients who were suffering from sudden death. Initial complainants, who included not only GPs, but funeral directors, and even taxi drivers, were rebuked, ignored, and even criticised for daring to make allegations about that fine upstanding member of the community. After he was rumbled, forensic examination of the computer records showed that Shipman had altered the medical record, *after* the death of his patient, to fit in with the story.

Why does accuracy matter? Because when a death is registered, the information is fed directly to the ONS – the Office of National Statistics. These figures are collated and end up in a report on causes of death in the UK. These figures are then often compared with other countries. A few years ago, there was quite a bit in the medical press about 'the French paradox'. If French people were smoking Gauloises, swigging gallons of red wine and feasting on foie gras, and cheese, and chocolate, why were they not dying of heart disease? Perhaps because French doctors were not putting 'heart attack' on the death certificate. They were allowed to put 'old age'.

And what of cremation? If the deceased is for cremation, the law requires that two doctors sign the necessary forms. Part 1 is usually signed by the doctor who signed the death certificate. Part 2 has to be signed by a doctor who is not in the same practice as the doctor who signed part 1. The doctor who signs part 2 is required to inspect the body. The form asks 'Did you inspect the body?' Response –*yes*. 'What sort of examination did you perform?' Response – *external*. In practice this means you went to the undertakers, they pulled out the drawer from the fridge, you checked the name tag on the foot, and made sure there wasn't a large knife sticking out of the chest. For *external* read *cursory*. Interestingly, Shipman made a great song and dance of this, studiously checking the body, even asking for it to be turned over. Thorough, you see.

Post- Shipman, the forms changed. The doctor doing part 2 is now required to question the doctor who did part 1, any nursing staff involved in the care of the patient, and the relatives of the deceased to ensure that they have no concerns about the mode of death. But you are entitled to put 'unable to contact' in the relatives section, and your conversation with doctor 1 does not have to be face-to-face. You ring them up.

'Ethel Smith, you have given *cardiopulmonary degeneration* as cause of death, tell me about her.'

'Well, as you can see, she was 91 years old, she had been failing for some time, I saw her at home the day before she died, and she was very weak. She passed away peacefully in the night.'

'OK, I'll fill in the form.'

You don't think Shipman could get round this?

Controlled drugs

Controlled drugs include things like pethidine and morphine and diamorphine (heroin). Because of the propensity for abuse, and because they can be dangerous drugs in their own right, their use is controlled. This means that they are kept in a locked cupboard, and that there is a register of their use. Pre-Shipman, the system allowed the GP to take a box of ampoules out of the cupboard, and enter into the log book '10 ampoules of pethidine 100mg to doctor's bag'. The remaining supplies had to tally with the written record. These 10 ampoules would then be used at the discretion of the doctor. As we have learned from Shipman, his discretion meant injecting most of it into himself. But he was caught, reformed, and allowed to return to general practice, where he now injected it into healthy, elderly people to kill them.

Post-Shipman, things tightened up, with the requirement to account for every ampoule of controlled drug, e.g. 100 mg pethidine administered to Mrs. Smith on 1.5.2010. But that does not necessarily mean that the pethidine arrived in Mrs. Smith. She might have received an injection of saline instead, allowing a dodgy doctor to accumulate a little supply of the good stuff for whatever evil purposes.

Revalidation

Whilst some form of revalidation for GPs had been mooted for some time, the Shipman case certainly accelerated its implementation. Revalidation 'is the process by which doctors demonstrate that they are up to date and fit to practice' according to the RCGP (Royal College of General Practitioners). In order to become revalidated, the GP has to undergo five annual 'appraisals.' This is a quite structured process. For each appraisal, the GP has to prepare a folder covering, among other things;

-personal development –how you saw yourself moving forward over the next year or two

-health and probity – whether you are still fit, physically, mentally and ethically

-cautions and criminal offences

-keeping up to date, a requirement to demonstrate at least 50 hours of learning, through journals, conferences, lectures etc.

-significant events – this might be a misdiagnosis, a death, a prescribing error

-feedback – from patients and colleagues, compliments and criticisms received

The culmination of all this was the appraisal interview, conducted by a fellow GP. This would last about half a day. I have to say, after initial misgivings, I quite enjoyed the whole process. How often do you get to spend several hours just talking about yourself, your job, your concerns? You could moan about Jeremy Hunt when he was Health secretary, you could moan about Jeremy Hunt when he wasn't Health secretary.

Towards the end of my general practice career, I started to take some liberties. The thank you cards from patients would be recycled year after year, any unfinished development plans would be relabelled 'work in progress'. My final appraisal came just weeks before my retirement date. My enthusiastic appraiser asked me 'Are there any patient groups that pose a particular challenge to your approach to practice?' I stared into the middle distance, affecting serious consideration, before replying 'Yes.

Scum'. The raised eyebrow indicated that this was not the expected, nor desired, response. I have to say that my answer was largely tongue-in-cheek, well, just a little bit, well, not at all, come to think of it.

'Would you care to elaborate?' Not so much a question as a directive.

'Well, you know, drug addicts who refuse to accept any help, who lie to you, deceive you, steal from old ladies to fund their habit. People who think the health service exists to serve them, even though they have trivial or imaginary complaints. People who are rude to me, to my staff, to the ambulance crews, the hospital staff. People who are aggressive, ignorant, abusive for no other reason than they think that everything that befalls them is unfair, and everyone else's fault but theirs. Whingers, idle, feckless, ungrateful, you know, scum.' (I was about to add Daily Mail readers, but felt that was a stretch too far).

Long pause.

'And do you think that you might need some form of re-training to enable you to overcome these difficulties, to reshape your attitudes?'

'No, I don't, because I feel sure that my sentiments are shared by a large number of health care staff, both here, and up and down the country, and I think it is the attitudes of others, including the scum and the whingers, that need reshaping.'

And I retire in a few weeks.

I passed my appraisal.

Don't get me wrong, I am a supporter of appraisal and revalidation, and felt that its introduction was long overdue. I feel that it does improve standards in general practice, and, in fact, contributes towards a profession that is better informed, better disciplined and, dare I say it, more content.

Will any of the above measures prevent another Shipman? No. You can't legislate against lunacy. So you will just have to be reassured that 99.99% of GPs are decent, hard-working, ethical, compassionate human beings who care about their patients, and who treasure the art of medicine.

Rare stuff

Medical textbooks, and in particular, books on general practice, are fond of pointing out the rarity, or relative probability of encountering, certain conditions and diseases. Thus you might find 'this abnormality occurs in 1 in every 10,000 births', or 'the average GP will see this disease about once every seven years or so'. Fine. You might be forgiven for failing to recognise Sotos syndrome (cerebral gigantism) as it is exceedingly rare. You would expect to be able to detect the tell-tale features of Down's syndrome in a newborn baby. Every now and then, you will astound your colleagues (and yourself) by making a brilliant diagnosis in a case which has confounded others. But there is one condition you hope never to meet, one condition where you dread missing the diagnosis, because the consequences are catastrophic, often fatal. I am talking about meningococcal meningitis, the very thought of which causes shivers down the spine of every parent whose child develops a rash. The condition is now more correctly referred to as 'meningococcal disease', as this term includes both the meningitis and the septicaemia which often accompanies it, a deadly combination.

Being a seaside town, each summer heralded the arrival of scores of foreign language students, mostly from Scandinavia. They would drift along the esplanade in clumps, identical blond teenagers in identical sweatshirts, carrying identical rucksacks. Convenient for the teachers charged with shepherding them to their various activities. Convenient also to chancers and pickpockets, as they were announcing to the world 'Hello, I am a foreigner in a foreign land, I'm vulnerable, and probably carrying a wad of cash around for essential purchases like candy floss, burgers, and tacky souvenirs'.

The parents of these children had been conned into parting with lots of hard-earned Krone, in the belief that little Hans or Gretel would be put up in a five star hotel, and fed fine cuisine. Not the case. They stayed for the most part with 'host families' – usually (but not always) hard up families who needed some extra cash. They in turn were paid a pathetically small amount to provide not only lodgings, but three meals a day, including a packed lunch. The balance between what the parents paid, and what the hosts earned, went to the company. Somebody, somewhere was making a nice little living out of this venture.

One morning, I was presented with a sullen, 14-year-old Swedish girl with amazingly long legs and amazingly short shorts. The 'host mother' seemed put out, as the rest of the group were on an outing to some castle, whereas she had to drag Lottie to see the doctor, as she had a headache and a temperature. I took a brief history, and checked the patient over. Nothing to find, except the fact that she was indeed flushed and hot. 'Probably a viral infection' I said 'take her home, let her rest in bed, give her fluids and paracetamol.' They turned to leave, and it was then that my sixth sense kicked in, and I decided to take a closer look at the bruise on Lottie's upper thigh. Surely not?....

I did the blanching test (pressing a glass against the bruise to see if it blanches and disappears – it did not), and checked for any other bruises or rashes – none. But she was clearly unwell. I called a colleague into the room for a second opinion, and we both stood their stroking our chins for a few seconds. I made my decision. 'I'm giving her the penicillin'. Not an easy choice, as the intramuscular injection of a large dose of penicillin, though potentially lifesaving, is famously painful. I then phoned the on-call paediatric doctor.

'Potential case of meningococcal disease' I stated confidently.

'Where is the patient as present?'

'Sitting here in front of me.'

'Is she conscious?'

'Yes.'

'And covered in a rash?'

'She has one lesion on her leg.'

I could almost picture the sneer on his face, almost hear the snort of derision, as he turned to his colleague and whispered 'Got a right one here.'

'Well, then, you had better send her in.'

159

The ambulance was called, and she was duly dispatched to the local hospital. I have to depend on eye-witness testimony for what happened next. She arrived at the nursing station, clutching my referral letter.

'So this is the meningococcal case, then?' queried the self-same cocky paediatric doctor. 'Perhaps she can *walk* to that bed over there so that I can assess her *properly*'.

At this exact point in time, Lottie complained of feeling dizzy. A wheelchair was produced, and she collapsed into it. As she was being wheeled down the ward, she became unconscious. The tell-tale blotches of meningococcal disease were marching up her arms and legs. Within minutes, she was in intensive care, covered in haemorrhages, on a drip and fighting for her life. She survived, miraculously without any of the complications that can ensue, like limb amputations. Her family flew over from Sweden, and came to see me in the surgery, to personally thank me for saving their daughter's life.

'Thank heavens you took the decision to give her penicillin' said my colleagues.

'Thank heavens she was wearing skimpy shorts' I thought. Had she been wearing jeans, she would be dead by now.

Of course, I took every opportunity to ring the paediatric doctor, to check on the progress of my patient. Not that I was rubbing his nose in it, you understand, and perhaps three phonecalls a day was a little over the top.

Two weeks later, I was called out at night to see a poorly toddler staying in a badly lit caravan in a field in the middle of nowhere. He had a fever, and a suspicious rash. He had actually been seen in the A and E department earlier that day, and sent away with Calpol and advice. I swallowed hard as I drew up the penicillin and calculated the dose. This time, my phonecall was more graciously accepted. The diagnosis was correct, and this child also survived.

Things occur in threes. My partner admitted a six month old baby a few weeks later with the same condition. Again, all was well. No connection was found between the cases, who were all visitors to the town from different parts of the globe. Neither of us knowingly saw another case in the rest of our careers.

Brenda Bolton was the sort of patient who seemed to spend as much time in the local hospital as in her own, overheated, cluttered flat. She was obese and a smoker. She suffered from COPD – chronic obstructive pulmonary disease. She had an array of inhalers which she kept on an overflowing tea tray, together with the rest of her medication, *Take a Break* magazine, and an ashtray which was whisked away as the doctor arrived, leaving behind its indelible pungent aroma of stale nicotine. She made frequent, usually unreasonable, and often irritating demands on the health service. She was known to every GP in town, every ambulance crew, and most of the doctors and nurses in the local hospital. Today was no exception. The call came in, I arrived to see her using her inhalers with all the technique of a bad actor pretending to have asthma in an episode of *Eastenders*. For all the good it was doing, she might as well have sprayed it around like a Glade air freshener.

'I'm really bad this time, doc, can't hardly breathe.'

'Well, I'll just set up the nebuliser, and see if that helps.'

Nebuliser set up, and an appropriate dose of two powerful medications wending their way in to the tar-clogged recesses of her diseased lungs.

'Not working, doc, I think I need to be in the ward.'

'I'm not sure that's necessary.' But I was already feeling that I was losing the battle, and previous experience had taught me that it would be futile to persist. Eventually, I rang the on-call doctor, who sighed sympathetically, and agreed her admission. I called for an ambulance, did not even need to give the address.

Whilst I was waiting, my bleep went off. A child in the next street with a bad cough. I phoned the mother.

'He's got a terrible cough, doc, started this morning. Sounds like he's got a really sore throat or something.'

I could hear something in the background, a sound that I had heard before, and didn't want to hear again.

'Is that him that I can hear in the room with you? Put the phone closer to him.'

I froze. This was not 'a bad cough'. The child had epiglottitis, and the awful raw sound was the results of his increasingly futile attempts to suck air through an opening which was getting narrower by the minute.

Epiglottitis is the swelling of the epiglottis, the flap at the base of the tongue which stops food going into the windpipe. Symptoms develop rapidly, with difficulty swallowing, drooling, and then difficulty breathing. Treatment often involves the insertion of an endotracheal tube to keep the airway open, together with antibiotics and steroids. The most important thing is to keep the child - and the parents - calm, as upset leads to crying, which aggravates the problem.

'I'll be straight there.' I then called the ambulance, and told them to divert Mrs. Bolton's van to the child's address.

'What's going on?' she demanded.

'Emergency.' I said, as I rushed out. *Real* emergency.

The child looked very ill, and was deteriorating. I was relieved to see the blue flashing light pull up outside the door. I travelled in the ambulance to the hospital, fully aware that I might need to put that tube into the child's narrow throat. I was met at the door of the hospital by the consultant paediatrician, and an anaesthetist, into whose expert care I transferred my patient.

I eventually returned to see Mrs. Bolton, who had improved and no longer needed an ambulance, if she had aver needed one at all. Still charged with adrenaline, I decided it was time to give her some lifestyle advice, which included smoking cessation, weight loss, and stopping wasting valuable NHS resources. It was harsh, and afterwards, I felt I had gone over the top. Some years later, I was attending a patient in a community centre in a nearby town. The receptionist stopped me and said 'You don't remember me, do you?' I peered closely. It was a slimmer, healthier, happier version of a woman I once knew as Brenda Bolton. 'That day you had a right go at me, I was furious at what you said. But I was also furious with myself for allowing myself to get into that state. I changed my life. I want to say thank you.'

We accept that not all of our advice to patients hits home. When it does, it makes everything worthwhile. Well, for a day or so.

Time to go

One evening in October 2013, most of the local GPs were at a meeting called by the Primary Care Trust (PCT). An eminent medical politician was to address us all on 'The Future of General Practice.'

His opening sentence did not inspire confidence.

'There is no good news.'

He went on to explain that the current government thinking was that they wanted GPs to be available, to provide medical services, from 8 a.m. to 8 p.m. This would be a contractual necessity.

Furthermore, the sanctity of the pension system was about to be breached, with a cap to be introduced on lifetime earnings, which would effectively reduce final pensions. This would prove to be counterproductive, as there would be little point in some clinicians continuing to work beyond a certain age, or, in the hospital setting, doing any overtime. This would, in turn, lead to a stampede out of the door, as GPs retired early, depleting a GP population which was already at crisis point. Well done, chaps.

There was further bad news on targets, the QOF, and working conditions. I scribbled something on my notepad, and passed it across the table to my partner.

'1.4.2015? What's that?'

'My retirement date.' I replied.

I had given them eighteen months' notice - much, much more than the requirement, as I knew they would struggle to recruit.

But there were other compelling reasons behind my decision.

It was becoming harder to keep up to date. *General* practice means just that – you have to be a *generalist*. That means knowing about asthma, heart disease, cancer, social care. It means keeping up to date with the latest research, the newest drugs, but also the changes in the law, the most recent and infuriating targets to be met, the algorithms, street drugs, the medicolegal situation, clinical governance, even trends on social media. I have to be honest and declare that it was a huge effort, and a battle that I felt I was just beginning to lose. In my book, it was not acceptable to keep walking down the corridor of the surgery to ask a younger, more up-to-date partner about that new inhaler, or whether I needed to do something about the teenager who had texted a picture of his willy to his girlfriend.

I also feared that I would become a negative influence on the workings of the practice. As senior partner, I was involved in all the decisions about the future, be it staffing levels, refurbishment of the waiting room, or whether we were going to agree to the latest strategy decision from the local Trust. Some of these decisions had financial implications, and, as someone who was approaching retirement, I had a large lump sum and a healthy pension to look forward to. I did not need to be scrabbling around for the latest £1 on offer for yet another form to be filled. But younger, poorer, hungrier partners might.

I had seen enough policy documents and NHS reorganisations over thirty years, to have developed a health cynicism, and it was all too easy to say 'we've already tried that' or 'we'll put the work in, then they will change it all again in six months.' A regular doom merchant. The young partners deserved the right to make their own decisions (and possible mistakes) about the future.

The threat of complaints and medicolegal action was undeniably a factor. I had made it through thirty years without a significant complaint. I had never had occasion to call upon the services of the Medical Protection Society, to whom I had cheerfully given a large chunk of my earnings over that period. The General Medical Council had never sent me a chilling letter in a crisp white envelope. My luck might run out. Not because I would become sloppy, and start making incorrect diagnoses, or because I would have a moral lapse, but because the culture had changed. Fuelled by the media, both conventional and social, GPs had become the target of compensation-obsessed patients and solicitors. This had brought about a change in practice, a defensiveness, which was not welcome. I had always been taught to record positives during an examination, and a negative finding if it was significant. So, an entry for a patient presenting with abdominal pain might once have read as 'tenderness *was* present in the upper abdomen. There was *no* distension.' But now it might read as 'tenderness *was* present in the upper abdomen. There was *no* distension. There were *no* varicose veins in the left leg. The right arm was *not* missing. The patient *was* alive.' You think I'm joking? Then take a look at the computer generated nonsense that masquerades as a discharge summary from A and E.

You have already had the benefit of my views on the changing philosophy of the NHS, and the target-driven culture, and pay for performance, but other things had changed as well. This is more controversial, but the sense of fun had gone. It was no longer acceptable to have banter with the receptionists. I am NOT talking #metoo stuff, I am not talking about misplaced sexual comments, just every day, jokey, witty, chat. Or even an innocent 'you look nice today'. And if your view is that 'this sort of behaviour' was never appropriate in the workplace, then I'm sorry, but I disagree, and so, as a matter of fact, do most of the female receptionists I have been fortunate to work with. Oh, and for the record, you don't look nice today.

It was time to go. But like previous honourable partners before me, I had decided to work with full commitment up to the last minute of the last day. No slacking off, no dodging meetings or responsibilities, no early finishes. And so it was that I saw my last patient at 5.50 p.m. on a Friday afternoon, did the necessary referral letter, cleared my desk and my folders, and walked away from general practice forever.

When I applied to this practice in 1985, I was one of a hundred hopefuls. Now, despite advertising the vacancy for six months, not just locally, but nationally, and even internationally, there were no applicants.

Not one.

Epilogue

This book opened with a quotation about 'the art of medicine'.

Medicine is indeed an art, and nowhere is this better exemplified than general practice. In addition to a phenomenal knowledge base encompassing anatomy, diseases, investigations, treatments and healthcare models, there is the requirement to keep up to date, to meet targets, to demonstrate probity.

But general practice is about listening. More than that, it is about *hearing* what the patient is telling you. An old maxim I encountered at medical school was 'listen to the patient, they are telling you the diagnosis.'

A few years ago, a general practice medical journal ran a competition to find the best maxim for successful practice. The winner was 'Never manhandle the man with his hand on the handle.' This pithy sentence refers to the reluctant male patient who is about to leave the room, when he turns and says 'there was something else, doctor....' This moment is pivotal, because he is about to divulge the real reason he came to see you, not the nonsense he has spent the last ten minutes telling you. My own maxim might have been 'seventeen-year-old girls never go to the doctor with a sore throat, but we see a lot of seventeen-year-old girls with sore throats.' It behoves the GP to see beneath the poorly constructed veneer and ask 'was there anything else?' 'Well, I was wondering about going on the pill....'

GPs are compassionate individuals. They care deeply about their patients, their lives, their suffering. If nothing else, they offer a kind word, a knowing look, a hand on the arm.

This is to be treasured, but it is at risk.

I am not a Luddite. I recognise the march of progress, the increasing complexity of care, the need for data, the need for evidence-based medicine, and the arguments for cost-effectiveness. But we are overrun with targets, algorithms, rules, restrictions. We are lorded over by managers who may be here today and gone tomorrow. Many medical conditions last for decades, yet governments are incapable of making decisions which last longer than a term in office. We need a strategic all-party, long term approach to healthcare. We need to find a solution to the exodus of GPs, we need to have a doctor / patient ratio that allows good practice, and facilitates training and recruitment.

When I entered medical school in 1974, the government had just published a report showing that 70% of the healthcare budget was spent in secondary care (hospitals) and 30% was spent in primary care (GPs). This was despite the fact that 70% of activity was carried out in primary care, and 30% in secondary care. This report set out ways to redress the balance. Forty-five years later, the figures are still the same.

We need change.

Amen.

How the years can slip away

How the years can slip away

Moment, weekend, decade, day

And yet the bonds we forge hold strong

To anchor us where we belong

A word, a sigh, a look, a touch

Despite the past could mean so much

A life less lived, a turning page

A pace, a race, a glimpse, an age

That brought us to this mirror'd day

Oh, how the years can slip away

How the years can slip away

For actors in a restless play

With lines half-learned, and timid air

A role too far, too pierced with care

Arranged, we wait each curtain's fall

The welcome night that hides us all

A shadowed smile, remembered kiss

Designed for us to end like this

New hearts to touch, too much to say

Oh, how the years can slip away.

Eugene Hughes, 2009.

Acknowledgements

I must thank the following individuals;

Neil M for his priceless advice on medicolegal matters

Pam B for reading the first draft, and her helpful suggestions

Pam S for correcting the spelling mistakes

John J for his funny contributions

Steve H for sorting out the cover photo

Jan G for being an unwitting model

.... and BH for being too afraid to read the first draft 'in case it was rubbish'

Printed in Great Britain
by Amazon